PRAISE FOR THE SEC
*B IS FOR B*
*12 STEPS TOWARD A*
*LIFE AT HOME A.*

"Whether you are a health care practitioner, attorney, CPA, or parent and home manager—regardless of your path—the pull of 24/7 access to technology and the fast pace of modern life can feel overwhelming. This book provides a holistic approach to finding your place of peace, purpose, and pleasure in an immensely readable and enlightening way. Follow Weinstein's 12-step approach and get started with improving your life!"

*–Kathryn Kadilak, MPA, BS*
*President, Innovative Workplace Strategies, and former*
*U.S. Department of Justice Work-Life Director*

"*B Is for Balance, Second Edition* is a treasure chest of wisdom insights that reminds us that energy and purpose management are the keys to health, vitality, and professional renewal. The 12-step blueprint for vitality proposed in this book is an invitation to remember and activate the essential requirements of healthy living. As nurses, when we care for ourselves, we are better able to care for others."

*–Daniel J. Pesut, PhD, RN, PMHCNS-BC, FAAN*
*Professor of Nursing Population Health and Systems Cooperative Unit*
*Director, Katharine Densford Center for International Nursing Leadership*
*Katherine R. and C. Walton Lillehei Chair in Nursing Leadership*
*University of Minnesota School of Nursing*

"*B Is for Balance* is a delightful, easy-to-read book that reminds us all that we do not live to work. In today's busy electronic world, it is refreshing to be reminded how to slow down, get in tune with our bodies, and enjoy life. This new edition addresses the very real problem of sleep deficits and the impact on our lives. Weinstein threads her grandchild throughout the book, giving examples of life through a child's eyes. Her book opens doors and lets us remember what it is like to be caught up in the wonder of life—not the busyness."

*–Carole Kenner, PhD, RN, FAAN*
*Carol Kuser Loser Dean/Professor*
*School of Nursing, Health and Exercise Science, The College of New Jersey*

# Copyright © 2015 by Sigma Theta Tau International

*The Honor Society of Nursing, Sigma Theta Tau International (STTI) is a nonprofit organization whose mission is to support the learning, knowledge, and professional development of nurses committed to making a difference in health worldwide. Founded in 1922, members include practicing nurses, instructors, researchers, policymakers, entrepreneurs and others. STTI's 494 chapters are located at 676 institutions of higher education throughout Australia, Botswana, Brazil, Canada, Colombia, Ghana, Hong Kong, Japan, Kenya, Malawi, Mexico, the Netherlands, Pakistan, Portugal, Singapore, South Africa, South Korea, Swaziland, Sweden, Taiwan, Tanzania, United Kingdom, United States, and Wales. More information about STTI can be found online at www.nursingsociety.org.*

Sigma Theta Tau International
550 West North Street
Indianapolis, IN, USA 46202

To order additional books, buy in bulk, or order for corporate use, contact Nursing Knowledge International at 888.NKI.4YOU (888.654.4968/US and Canada) or +1.317.634.8171 (outside US and Canada).

To request a review copy for course adoption, email solutions@nursingknowledge.org or call 888. NKI.4YOU (888.654.4968/US and Canada) or +1.317.634.8171 (outside US and Canada).

To request author information, or for speaker or other media requests, contact Marketing, the Honor Society of Nursing, Sigma Theta Tau International at 888.634.7575 (US and Canada) or +1.317.634.8171 (outside US and Canada).

**ISBN: 9781938835841**
**EPUB ISBN: 9781938835858**
**PDF ISBN: 9781938835865**
**MOBI ISBN: 9781938835872**

---

Library of Congress Cataloging-in-Publication Data

Weinstein, Sharon, author.
 B is for balance : 12 steps toward a more balanced life at home and at work / Sharon M. Weinstein. -- Second edition.
  p. ; cm.
 Includes bibliographical references and index.
 ISBN 978-1-938835-84-1 (alk. paper) -- ISBN 978-1-938835-85-8 (ePUB) -- ISBN 978-1-938835-86-5 (PDF) -- ISBN  978-1-938835-87-2 (Mobi)
 I. Title.
 [DNLM: 1.  Nurses--psychology. 2.  Burnout, Professional--prevention & control. 3.  Nurse's Role--psychology. 4.  Quality of Life. 5.  Workload--psychology. WY 87]
 RT82
 610.7306'9--dc23
                        2014026994

---

First Printing, 2014

**Publisher:** Dustin Sullivan

**Acquisitions Editor:** Emily Hatch

**Editorial Coordinator:** Paula Jeffers

**Cover Designer:** Rebecca Batchelor

**Interior Design/Page Layout:** Rebecca Batchelor

**Principal Book Editor:** Carla Hall

**Development and Project Editor:** Kevin Kent

**Copy Editor:** Charlotte Kughen

**Proofreader:** Barbara Bennett

**Indexer:** Joy Dean Lee

# DEDICATION

A mom, wife, educator, speaker, author, coach, clinician, international consultant, I lived a life that others dreamed about—and all of the pieces seemed to fit. You might be asking, "How is that possible with so many titles, so much to do, and so little time?"

I knew that I could not maintain the pace that I had created, often working 100 hours weekly, sometimes 3 countries per week, and I knew that I needed to shift my paradigm. And, I did!

It was becoming a grandmother that opened my eyes to life as a balancing act, and what it could do for me and others! To my grandchildren—for creating a level of awareness in me that I have come to love and enjoy, each and every day!

SMW

# ACKNOWLEDGMENTS

By all means, while you're changing the world, don't forget about the everyday human needs of those whose lives you touch. I am certainly well aware of those who have helped me to realize my own dreams:

My husband Steve, who taught me that I could be anything I set my mind to be.

My family, for their constant belief in me and in my ability to be all things to all people!

A special thank-you to the team of professionals from Sigma Theta Tau, including Emily Hatch, acquisitions editor; Kevin Kent, project and development editor; Charlotte Kughen, copy editor; and Barbara Bennett, proofreader. Thanks to Joy Dean Lee, for expert indexing of the manuscript. The cover provides a clear message, and it is a reflection of this second edition of *B Is for Balance*. Thanks to Rebecca Batchelor, who provided a cover design that truly depicts the concept of achieving balance in one's life at home and at work. And, finally, thanks to the contributing authors, Dr. Marla Vannucci and Debbie Reynolds Hughes, each of whom has found balance in her life and shares the model with clients each and every day; they now share their message with you, the reading audience. These are lessons learned from those who have lived them.

# About the Authors

Led by Sharon Weinstein, the author team combines the talents and wellness perspectives of three seasoned leaders with a powerful background in practice, process, holistic health, psychology, and education.

## Sharon M. Weinstein, MS, RN, CRNI, FACW, FAAN

President and founder of SMW Group LLC, Core Consulting Group, and the Global Education Development Institute, Weinstein is the author of nine texts and more than 160 peer-reviewed publications. Recent publications include *Plumer's Principles and Practice of Infusion Therapy* (9th ed.) with Mary Hagle and *Nursing without Borders: Values, Wisdom, and Success Markers*, co-edited with Ann Marie T. Brooks. Upcoming publications include *Side by Side*, *Connectivity*, and *From Learn to Type to Learn to Live*. A member of the National Wellness Institute, Infinity Foundation, Chicago Healers, the American College of Wellness, the American Nurses Association, and the American Holistic Nurses Association, Weinstein has been seen on NBC 5 Chicago and other media outlets on topics including attitude, balance, healthy schools, believing in oneself, EMF sensitivity, and adrenal fatigue.

Weinstein earned her spot as the go-to professional for education, resources, well-being, and work/life balance. Weinstein draws on her own life experiences to help others discover their life's purpose. She is the founder of the Integrative Health Forum (IHF, www.ihfglobal.com), an interdisciplinary alliance of licensed healthcare professionals whose mission is to serve the professionals and associations that promote health and well-being in individuals, organizations, and communities around the globe. She is an independent founding member of Alphay, a global health and wellness company.

Weinstein has been actively involved in Sigma Theta Tau International and recently championed the creation of the first chapter in the Republic of Armenia; she is a member of the Alpha Lambda chapter. Recently elected to a leadership role within the American Holistic Nurses Association (AHNA) and to the board of directors of the National Speakers Association (NSA), she is past president of the Infusion Nurses Society (INS) and past chair of the Infusion Nurses Certification Corporation (INCC). Weinstein serves as a member of the Expert Panel on Global Nursing/ American Academy of Nursing.

She earned a master's degree in health management and gerontology from North Texas State University, a certificate in health administration from Trinity University, a bachelor's degree in nursing and behavioral science from Wilmington College, and a diploma from Pennsylvania Hospital School of Nursing. She is a graduate of the Kellogg School of Management's Executive Management Program, a fellow of the American College of Wellness, a fellow of the American Academy of Nursing, and adjunct clinical professor at the University of Illinois Chicago, College of Nursing. Weinstein is a member of the National Speakers Association (NSA). Her research interests include workplace wellness, fatigue, and longevity. Wellness is what she does!

## DEBBIE REYNOLDS HUGHES, MSN, FNP, PMHNP, BC

Hughes, a dually certified nurse practitioner in family medical and psychiatric mental health, offers patients a holistic approach to healthcare. She received her master of science degree from the University of Nebraska Medical Center in a dual-track program that emphasized holistic care by simultaneously treating the patient's physical and psychological health. As a holistic practitioner, Hughes's expertise in psychiatry, functional medicine, nutrition, bio-identical hormones, and anti-aging medicine guides patients to experience total health using the most effective protocols. She has worked in the medical field for more than 30 years in a variety of settings, including hospital medical/surgical units, home and community health, public schools, long-term care, and most recently private practice. In 2006, she founded Holistic Harmony Healthcare, a corporation committed to providing holistic comprehensive care and wellness. She is board certified by the American Nurses Credentialing Center as a Psychiatric

Mental Health Nurse Practitioner and also with the American Academy of Nurse Practitioners as a Family Nurse Practitioner. She is also board certified in functional and anti-aging medicine through the American Academy of Anti-Aging Medicine. Hughes is a member of the American Nurses Association, American Academy of Nurse Practitioners, American Holistic Nurses Association, Nebraska Nurse Practitioners, and American Academy of Anti-Aging Medicine.

## Marla Vannucci, PhD

Marla Vannucci, PhD, is a licensed clinical psychologist in private practice and an associate professor at the Adler School of Professional Psychology. She received her MA and PhD in Counseling Psychology from Northwestern University, and her BA in psychology from New York University. She has worked in a variety of clinical settings, including college counseling, community mental health, inpatient psychiatric, hospital/primary care, residential, and private practice. Her clinical specialties include couples therapy, parenting, trauma, and workplace wellness. In addition, Vannucci brings expertise in organizational development and consultation. Previously, as a senior consultant at Deloitte & Touche Tohmatsu, her consulting engagements included employee wellness program design, leadership training and coaching, and institutional assessment. Prior to joining Adler, Vannucci served as the director of clinical services at the Chicago School of Professional Psychology, where she oversaw the design and management of student wellness programs, and served as training director for advanced clinical training programs. Vannucci's ongoing research explores supervision, mentorship, and student learning. Vannucci is a Certified Positive Discipline Parent and Teacher Educator, as well as a Certified Freedom from Smoking Program Facilitator. She has been featured in *The Economist*, Foxnews.com, and on Chicago Public Radio, discussing issues such as parenting, social media, consumer behavior, and disaster response. Vannucci would like to thank Abigail Damsky Brown for her research assistance and Kurt Vannucci for inspiring her to be present in life and for his love, support, and assistance in research related to mindfulness, flow, and engagement.

# TABLE OF CONTENTS

ABOUT THE AUTHORS                                    VII
FOREWORD                                             XIII
PREFACE TO THE SECOND EDITION                        XVII
INTRODUCTION                                         XIX

PART I  BALANCING BY KNOWING AND
        APPRECIATING SELF                            1

  1.  Knowing Your Purpose                           3
      By Debbie Reynolds Hughes

  2.  Simplify Your Life                             25
      By Sharon M. Weinstein

  3.  The Wages of Stress                            45
      By Sharon M. Weinstein

  4.  Focus and Begin to Dream Again                 67
      By Sharon M. Weinstein

  5.  Get Engaged...In Your Life                     91
      By Marla J. Vannucci

  6.  Putting Technology in Its Place: The Effect
      of Connectivity and Social Media              117
      By Sharon M. Weinstein

PART II FINDING AND KEEPING BALANCE                 141

  7   Fatigue                                        143
      By Sharon M. Weinstein

  8   Workplace Balance                              171
      By Sharon M. Weinstein

  9   Sleepless, and Not Just in Seattle             191
      By Sharon M. Weinstein

10  Be Happy, Eat Well, Get Moving,
    Live Longer, and Live Well                    211
    *By Sharon M. Weinstein*

11  Reinventing Yourself: Becoming More
    of You                                        243
    *By Sharon M. Weinstein*

12  Destiny in the Balance                        269
    *By Sharon M. Weinstein*

    26 Principles of Life                         285
    Index                                         291

# Foreword

We have entered a new era of how we think about life balance, health, and well-being. The fast pace of daily life, lack of exercise, poor food choices, and environmental risk factors are being recognized as factors in stress and disease. Each of us has the requisite capacity for achieving balanced integration of our human potentials. *B is for Balance: 12 Steps Toward a More Balanced Life at Home and at Work* offers many opportunities for self-reflection, self-assessment, self-evaluation, and self-care; it provides the framework for how to gain access to inner wisdom and intuition and apply it in our daily lives. As we take responsibility for making effective choices and changes in our lives, we place ourselves in a better position to clarify our life patterns, purposes, and processes.

How do you define health and wellness? *Health* is a person's experience of a sense of well-being, harmony, and unity. It includes honoring health beliefs, values, and one's worldview. It is a process of opening and widening personal awareness and consciousness to new possibilities. *Wellness* is becoming aware of how to reach our highest potential. In order to increase states of health and wellness, we can make wise choices and decisions about how we reduce risks factors that lead to disease, illness, and injuries (Dossey, Luck, & Schaub, 2014).

Today we recognize that life's balance, health, and well-being are a discovery process to be more creative, more resilient, more hardy, and to learn how to reduce anxiety and fear around life's challenges, as well as when confronted with chronic disease and stress-related illnesses (Dossey, B. M., 2013). Health and wellness require that we recognize that life is a continual change process, and as we reflect on life's meaning and purpose, that leads to healing. *Healing* is a process of understanding and integrating the many aspects of self, connecting to our inner wisdom, and embodying this daily in a way that results in balance and wholeness.

As we take time to enter into balance and harmony each day, our consciousness—our capacity to react to, attend to, and be aware of self and others—is enhanced. Consciousness subsumes all categories of experience, including perception, cognition, intuition, instinct, will, and emotion, at all levels. This includes those commonly termed "conscious," "subconscious," "superconscious," "unconscious," "intention," and "attention," without presumption of specific psychological or physiological mechanisms (Dossey, L., 2013).

Raising our consciousness is not a concept or a random technique someone thought up for self-improvement. Rather, it is a basic principle of how to be a human being and experience the integration of body, mind, and spirit. As we explore the foundations for balance, health, and healing, we mature and exercise our human capacity to go beyond individual identity and evolve to our highest potential, the transpersonal self. Understanding the dimensions of the transpersonal self is a major force leading to our daily balance. Yet, knowing states of the transpersonal self is not an end point, but a continuing, never-ending process.

We are able to be self-reflective, and this opens us to the experience of something greater than one's individual self. An impressive body of evidence reveals that consciousness is *nonlocal*—that is, it is not confined or localized to specific points in space, such as brains or bodies, nor localized or limited to specific points in time, such as the present (Dossey, L., 2013). The emerging picture of consciousness is that it has no spatial and temporal boundaries or limits. As such it is *infinite* in space and time, therefore immortal, omnipresent, and, ultimately, one. Thus, our consciousness has transpersonal dimensions. "Transpersonal" implies a personal understanding that is based on one's experiences of temporarily transcending or moving beyond one's usual identification with the limited biological, historical, cultural, and personal self at the deepest and most profound levels of experience possible. These ordinary ways of experiencing the self are recognized as an important but only a partial manifestation or expression of this much greater aspect of our being, including an expanded concept of our origin and destiny. It is a majestic vision of who we are that transcends the limits and boundaries of the individual self or ego. This recognition is empowering; it makes it more likely that we can achieve the balance and harmony that are Weinstein's premise in this remarkable book.

So, in order to achieve balance in life, it is useful to explore our worldview. A worldview includes that set of beliefs each of us holds about how the world operates, why things happen the way they do, the rules they follow, and how we fit into these patterns. We usually ignore what our worldview actually is, but it is invariably a powerful, guiding force in each of our lives. We cannot escape the effects of our worldview. We put our worldview into action as we begin each day with family, significant others, pets, entering the workplace, and so forth. Do we believe that we have control over our life or do things happen by? What is the purpose or meaning behind myriad events that emerge each day? Do we have choice in health and illness, or is our body entirely "on automatic"? Our worldview is a source of answers to these complex questions. The more conscious we become of the assumptions we make about our worldview and "how things work," the more effective we will become in our interactions with self and others—and the more likely we will be to achieve the balance that is this book's theme.

How can you become more conscious about your worldview and your choices in life? To be present for yourself or another, you must honor your personal needs or you will risk becoming a physical and emotional wreck. What are the current circumstances in your life? What are you willing to accept, and what should you consider changing? In the pages that follow, you will learn to cease obsessing about the things over which you have no control. You'll learn to honor yourself each day with a variety of strategies such as relaxation, imagery, music, meditation, or prayer. You'll see the value of creating an exercise program, taking relaxing and energizing hot baths or showers, eating nutritious foods, eliminating excess caffeine or junk food, exploring your dreams, and asking others for help when it's needed. You'll learn to honor your effort by telling yourself over and over what a good job you are doing, and repeating it until you believe it.

Bridges can be created between different persons that are transpersonal, as with distant healing intentions, intercessory prayer, shamanic healing, so-called miracles, and emotions such as love, empathy, and compassion. These approaches involve profound transpersonal experiences of being. They elevate our experiences outside our local self and ego. Through self-reflection, we deepen our capacity for healing—that lifelong journey into wholeness, out of which harmony and balance can grow in our relations with our family, our community, and all sentient life.

of Canada in 1909). I was intrigued by the cultural nuances everywhere I visited and the ability to meet my foreign nurse colleagues on a personal level, learning about their families, their education, and their vision for the future. My international work allowed me to appreciate human potential like never before. While I continually developed my own potential, I also continually thought, "What if?"

That "what if" involved the simple word *balance*; mine was nonexistent. As a person who has reinvented herself professionally throughout my career, I am aware of the challenges of work/life balance. Regardless of the association, clinical, or academic situation in which I found myself, I knew that something was missing...and that something was often at the expense of family relationships. Balancing a career or business with your personal life can be challenging, but it's not impossible. *B Is for Balance* sets the theme for a course of actions to build the life and career you want, need, and deserve. What better time to start that journey than now?

This book is about the countless number of professionals who walk the walk and talk the talk toward a balanced life. I transitioned toward a balanced life with support from my colleagues, mentors, and friends. I transitioned toward a balanced life through the love of my family. Like a house that cannot stand without a good foundation, my foundation is a balanced lifestyle.

Everything in life is a choice. You have to realize that you have chosen the life you are living right now. You pursue your dreams, and along that journey, you are forced to make many choices. This is perhaps life's greatest truth and most difficult lesson. It is what gives you the power to be yourself and to live the life you imagined. Don't allow self-doubt to interfere with your success or with the balanced life that you deserve. There is no such thing as an impossible dream; there are only dreams without action steps to make them a reality. Go ahead and dream those lofty dreams...and become them!

# INTRODUCTION

What is this thing called balance? You hear about it everywhere; you read about it; and you long for it. But what *is* it? What does it look like? Is it possible for normal people with jobs, families, hobbies, and multiple internal and external commitments to achieve balance in the modern world? The last answer is, of course, a resounding *yes*!

For most people, a balanced life means having optimal time to give to their families, their work, their communities, and their extracurricular activities. It also means enough money or compensation to be able to meet all the basic needs of existence and to save for future needs and desires. For most people, work consumes the majority of their days, and they have to fit in family, shopping for and preparing food, and more into their remaining time. Diet and optimal sleep frequently suffer when people are trying to do everything they need or want to do in a limited amount of "free" time. Relationships also suffer.

Nurses and other healthcare professionals know about balance and are the first to encourage their patients and clients to find balance in their lives. Unfortunately, nurses and healthcare professionals frequently find themselves doing the opposite of what they recommend: They work too much; they don't eat well; they sleep too little; they don't exercise; and they don't slow down when they get sick. There's always too much to do—too much at home, at work, at the kids' schools—for our training and education endeavors, and for our personal and professional goals.

Although it seems a daunting task to slow down enough to consider and contemplate achieving balance, it is a task worth doing—one that will improve your life in expected ways, but also in ways that may surprise you.

## BENEFITS OF ACHIEVING BALANCE

Achieving balance in your life can bring you amazing rewards. You can expect some or all of the following changes and improvements in your life as you move into balance:

- Improved health, including lower blood pressure and cholesterol levels
- Less stress and more happiness
- More energy
- Improved quality of life
- Better relationships
- Improved concentration
- More free time
- Potentially longer lifespan
- Sustainable health
- Simplicity in your life

## HOW THIS BOOK CAN HELP YOU ACHIEVE BALANCE

This book was written for all learning audiences to facilitate balancing their work and home lives. It is an active book. Although we give you sufficient information, anecdotes, and wisdom to inform your work, the goal is to move you into balance. Some of the features to help you in the goal are:

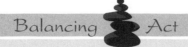

Balancing Act

Look for *Balancing Act* boxes to help you move forward in balancing your life. These exercises can be either cognitive or physical.

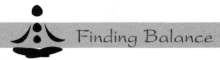
Finding Balance

*Finding Balance* boxes are at the end of each chapter. These exercises reinforce the message of the chapter and support your move toward a balanced life.

## REFERENCES

You will find references for further reading at the end of each chapter to help you explore specific topics in more detail.

# RECOVERING YOUR BALANCE

The challenge for all of us is to truly create balance in our lives, given the limitations of time and money freedom. It is a significant commitment to take the first steps toward recovering your balance in life, but those steps will reward you and your family many times over the actual investment.

Balance is an idea, to be sure, and while you might be able to find an app to address the topic, that app will not allow you to program balance into your life. The good news is that balance is within reach; it's just up to you to create it. The exercises in this book are not difficult. The difficulty lies in the commitment it takes to retake control of your life. Read on and begin the journey toward your own personal balance.

# PART I
## BALANCING BY KNOWING AND APPRECIATING SELF

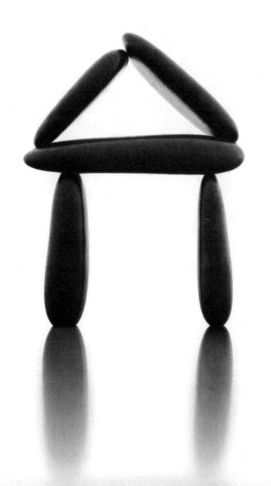

*"The purpose of life is to live a life of purpose."*

—Robert Bryne

# 1

# KNOWING YOUR PURPOSE

*—Debbie Reynolds Hughes, MSN, FNP, PMHNP, BC*

Every one of us wants to believe our lives are meaningful and that at the end of our lives we will have had a positive effect on the world. We seek meaning—physically, emotionally, and spiritually—through our work, our families, and our communities. This chapter helps you identify people who have been very influential in your life, list their qualities, and define who you want to be, what you want to experience, or what kind of results you want to realize, emotionally, financially, and materially. Something new in this edition is a look at the bucket list and how it affects who and what we are. The chapter also examines the happiness plan and four agreements to live a content, happy life and describes the purpose formula, which is the sum of values, strengths, and passions to identify your purpose. The chapter offers additional questions that help you express your purpose and then explore your alignment with that purpose. Your actions need to reflect your desired purpose in life. If it is my life purpose to live as healthy as I possibly can and be a great health role model and I still smoke, that is not being in alignment with my purpose.

# WHY AM I HERE?

Life purpose does not equate to only our work lives, nor is it simply our home lives or our roles within our families and communities. It is a combination—a balance, if you will—of all aspects of our lives that creates fulfillment. Life purpose is what gives meaning to our lives. It makes us feel alive, empowered, capable, and strong.

The fortunate among us discover our life purpose. This chapter presents clear and simple ways for you to identify your life purpose and prepare yourself for living out that purpose. After you have established your life purpose, you can be one of those fortunate individuals who know the answer to the question, "Why am I here?"

# WHY IDENTIFY YOUR LIFE PURPOSE?

1. It gives meaning to everything you do.
2. It directs and guides you.
3. It motivates you.

You are reading this book, and that means you are looking to achieve balance in your life. To find that balance, you must first find your center of knowing. You must know who you really are and what you really like. Meditation will help you develop the intuition necessary for finding your purpose, and finding your purpose will give you the center necessary for achieving balance. You cannot read about your intuition, listen to someone telling you what to do, or do anything other than discover the purpose of your life on your own.

*"At the center of your being you have the answer; you know who you are and you know what you want."*

*—Lao Tzu*

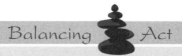

Balancing Act

# A SIMPLE APPROACH TO FINDING YOUR LIFE PURPOSE

If you want to discover your true purpose in life, you must first empty your mind of all the false perceptions you've been taught (including the idea that you may have no purpose at all).

So, how do you discover your purpose in life? Although there are many ways to do this—some of which are fairly involved—here is one of the simplest that anyone can do. The more open you are to this process, the faster it will work for you. Having doubts about it won't prevent it from working as long as you stick with it. It may just take longer to converge into meaningful insight.

# HERE'S WHAT TO DO:

Take out a blank sheet of paper or log onto your computer and open a blank document. The latter is faster, but writing manually helps some people. Choose the approach that will help you persist in the exercise.

- Write at the top, "What is my true purpose in life?"

- Write an answer (any answer) that pops into your head. It doesn't have to be a complete sentence. A short phrase is fine.

- Repeat the preceding step until you write the answer that makes you cry. This is your purpose.

That's it. It doesn't matter if you're a nurse, counselor, engineer, or a bodybuilder. It should take about 15 to 20 minutes to clear your head of all the clutter and the social conditioning about what you think your purpose in life is. You'll write down false answers that will come from your mind and your memories, but when the true answer finally arrives, it will feel like it's coming to you from a different source entirely.

For those who are entrenched in low-awareness living, you might need more time (possibly more than an hour) to get all the false answers out. If you persist, though, after 100 or 200 or maybe even 500 answers, you'll be struck by the answer that causes you to surge with emotion. That's the answer that comes from the heart.

As you go through this process, some of your answers will be similar. Then you might head off on a new tangent and generate 10 or 20 more answers with some other theme. That's fine. You can list whatever answers pop into your head as long as you just keep writing.

You may also discover a few answers that seem to give you a mini-surge of emotion, but they don't quite make you cry—they're just a bit off. Highlight those answers as you go along so you can come back to them to generate new permutations. Each of those answers reflects a piece of your purpose, but individually they aren't complete. When you start getting these kinds of answers, it means you're getting close to the real answer. Keep going.

When I did this exercise, it took me about 30 minutes and 93 steps to reach my final answer. When I felt resistance part of the way through the activity, I took a break, closed my eyes, meditated, and cleared my mind. This break helped me refocus, and the answers I received after began to have greater clarity. My final answer was, *"To live consciously and courageously, to resonate with love and compassion, guiding others on a path of well-being, and to leave this world in peace knowing I have experienced a life well lived."*

When you find your own unique answer to the question of why you're here, you will feel it resonate with you deeply. The words will seem to have a special energy and you will feel that energy whenever you read them.

Discovering your purpose is the easy part. The hard part is keeping it with you on a daily basis and working on yourself to the point where you achieve that purpose. I carry a copy of my purpose with me wherever I go, and I repeat it daily.

If you're inclined to question why and how the process works, wait until you have completed it yourself. Once you've done that, you'll have your own answer. This process works if you keep going until you reach convergence of ideas into insight. Usually, 80 to 90% of people achieve convergence in less than an hour. Give it a shot! You have everything to gain, and nothing to lose.

*Ask yourself…What gives your life meaning?*

# SELF-KNOWLEDGE

After you've identified your life purpose—or are working hard on it—it's important to learn more about yourself, including your habits, strengths, and weaknesses. In philosophy, *self-knowledge* commonly refers to knowledge of one's particular mental/spiritual states, including one's beliefs, desires, and sensations. If you have true friends, you have an important source of knowledge about things they have observed in you. Keep your friends close while you are identifying your life purpose and seeking self-knowledge. Talk with them about your exploration and ask for their support through input and kind reflection of their knowledge of your habits, strengths, and weaknesses. Seek input only from friends whom you trust completely. Remember, though, no one knows you better than you, so always be true to yourself and trust in your inner knowing.

At least since Descartes, most philosophers have believed that self-knowledge is importantly different from knowledge of the world external to oneself, including others' thoughts. Mindfulness—which is paying attention to one's current experience in a nonjudgmental way—helps us to learn more about our own personalities. Erika Carlson (2013), a psychology scientist at Washington University in St. Louis, reports that the components of mindfulness, attention, and nonjudgmental observation can overcome the major barriers to knowing ourselves. Practice these mindfulness techniques every day and ask yourself, "What do you love and what do other people say you are good at?"

"It is a sad fate for a man to die too well known to everybody else, and still unknown to himself."

—Francis Bacon

# IDENTIFY YOUR INFLUENTIAL PEOPLE

Influential people are leaders who have the characteristics of vision, courage, persistence, confidence, generosity, integrity, creativity, enthusiasm, character, and virtue. They have the ability to retain these qualities in the midst of chaos, confusion, and difficulty. They are extraordinary, and their presence energizes and inspires people. They rarely criticize anything or anyone because they are too busy fulfilling their purpose and getting the job done. They can be a grandparent, parent, friend, business contact, professional colleague, supervisor, or complete stranger.

Identifying influential people is important because you can learn and grow from their strength of character and purpose. Victor Frankl (1977) has been influential in the lives of many. From Frankl's experiences in concentration camps during World War II, including Auschwitz and Dachau, he observed that life has meaning under all conditions and that it is psychologically damaging when a person's meaning in life is blocked. In his book, *Man's Search for Meaning*, Frankl wrote that it is possible to find meaning in suffering.

"Fundamentally, therefore, any man can, even under such circumstances, decide what shall become of him—mentally and spiritually. He may retain his human dignity even in a concentration camp."

–Victor Frankl

Frankl's recommendation was to let life question you. What he meant is that life questions us through circumstances such as terminal diseases, divorce, and the death of loved ones. He believed that we benefit from crises in that we are forced to let go of petty concerns, conflicts, and the need for control. Even small crises can inform our days and our purpose. What did that near-miss car accident at the intersection this morning tell you? Were you rushing? Not paying attention? How would the difference of a few seconds one way or the other have changed your day or your life—in the short or long term? What about someone you just met who makes you think of someone in your life, past or present? How does that contact, the thoughts or questions arising from that contact, bring new or different meaning to your life?

Seek out influential people whose work speaks to your core beliefs and life purpose. Study their lives, their choices, and take strength from their struggles to fulfill their life work. Go back in history or go forward. Even children can be role models, reminding us of what really matters in life.

Think about some of the most famous influential people who have changed the way you view the world: Albert Einstein, Martin Luther King, Jr., Gandhi, and Florence Nightingale might be some examples. Write your own list of people who have influenced your life because of their passion.

Work to emulate the person who influences and inspires you and develop those qualities and behaviors that you recognize as important. Be a leader, and do not be afraid to show your authentic self. Dare to live the life most people only dream about. Think of Albert Einstein's words when you meet criticism: "Great spirits have always encountered violent opposition from mediocre minds."

## CONSIDER YOUR BUCKET LIST

The *bucket list* is a term coined by screenwriter Justin Jackham in an American comedy-drama film produced by Zadan and Meron (2007) and starring Jack Nicholson and Morgan Freeman. The main plot follows two terminally ill men on a road trip as they try to do everything on their wish lists before they "kick the bucket." Creating a bucket list can become a blueprint for a more fulfilling life. People don't realize that it is not just associated with dying; having a bucket list is actually a "way to live." What would be on your list?

If you'd like to make a bucket list that changes your life, use the following steps to make it happen:

1. Give yourself permission to dream big and be inspired. Keep thinking about it and talk to other people or look at others' lists for inspiration. Reading other people's bucket lists can stir desires you never knew you had.

2. Be specific. Choose items so specific and possible that you can visualize them happening. The subconscious mind doesn't know the difference between visualizing something and actually doing it.

3. Build in accountability. Sharing your list, whether online or just by talking about it, helps you become accountable for making progress toward your goals. Accountability increases your odds of success.

If you make your bucket list public knowledge and have people to hold you accountable, you are much more likely to accomplish the goals on your list. This is how I hold myself accountable, and I encourage you to share your bucket list.

A bucket list should be a work in progress; having one gives you something to strive for. The following are a few examples from my bucket list:

- Write a book on holistic health.
- Expand my corporation, Holistic Harmony Healthcare, to several locations.
- Travel to every continent in the world.
- Travel to every state in the United States. (I have a good start on this one.)
- Incorporate a yoga studio and nutrition bar within Holistic Harmony Healthcare.
- Develop more intuition and self-awareness.

Ask yourself…What do you notice as the main themes in your life?

## TRUST YOUR INTUITION

To discover your purpose, you must trust your intuition—which is the inner voice that leads to passion. It is a sixth sense independent of conscious reasoning. Sometimes, you cannot explain how you "know" something; you just know it. Most people know how to get what they *think* they want, but many do not *know* what they want.

The key to acting *on purpose* is to bring together the needs of the world with your unique gifts and talents. Working on purpose gives you a sense of direction. Life purpose comes from within and expresses itself in almost every aspect of life. The more you are in touch with your life purpose, the more you will notice how it drives you as an internally motivating factor to achieve your dreams.

To heighten your intuitiveness, you must first be aware of your needs. Psychologist Abraham Maslow (1943) described the fundamental human needs into a hierarchy. The most basic needs are physiological and safety. First, he argued, we must meet our physiological needs—oxygen, nutrition, and sleep—and feel secure. When physiological and safety needs are met, emotional needs—love and affection—are addressed. Next, Maslow concluded, even if physical, safety, and emotional needs are met, a discontentment and restlessness will soon develop unless we are doing what we are passionate about—in other words, unless we are fulfilling our higher needs or purpose. Finally, to feel ultimate peace, we must listen to our inner calling. This is what Maslow referred to as self-actualization. At this highest level, we live with purpose. This is the level at which those people who seek to emulate lives of service modeled by Nightingale, Gandhi, Nelson Mandela, and Mother Teresa operate so effectively.

Psychologist Clayton Alderfer (1972) compressed Maslow's five levels into three, known as the Existence/Relatedness/Growth (ERG) Theory:

1. **Existence:** Physiological and safety needs, such as hunger, thirst, and sex
2. **Relatedness:** External esteem—involvement with family, friends and co-workers
3. **Growth:** Internal esteem and self-actualization—desire for creativity and meaning

Alderfer designed his theory to be less rigid than Maslow's and used his model in organizational settings to help promote productivity and job satisfaction among employees. According to ERG, needs can be pursued simultaneously and in any order. He argues that people who can't meet their growth needs will revert to relationships to have their needs satisfied or will do no more than exist. If you are in the existence mode of living, there isn't much quality of life or job satisfaction.

When considering your needs, remember that everything in life is a choice. Remembering this truth causes you to realize that you have chosen the life you are living right now. You choose the food you eat, the clothes you wear, and most importantly, the thoughts you think. You are moving toward your purpose from birth to death and are forced to make choices along the way. This is life's greatest truth and most difficult lesson. Understanding this gives you the power to be yourself and live the life you have imagined. As you develop your intuitiveness, you will grow in the self-awareness that you have been living the life of your choice up to this point, and you have the freedom to change your life going forward.

*Ask yourself…What contribution do you want to make during your lifetime?*

# REIMAGINE YOUR LIFE PURPOSE

I want you to start this section with a visualization exercise—vividly picture the day of your funeral. What do you want to be said in your eulogy? What would your lifetime achievements be? What would matter the most at the end of your life? Is it what you are doing right *now*?

At the beginning of this chapter you were encouraged to list your passions—the things that make you cry. These are the things that matter most to you at the end of your life. Relationships, meaningful work, enjoying the beauty of nature—whatever it is that turns you on inside is what is going to make you feel fulfilled at the end of your life.

My passion evolves as I get older and is a result of loving life and my desire to serve others. In all that I do, I focus on my passion! Your passion can become your strength that drives you. Some people feel lost when asked what drives them. Open yourself up to true emotion and start to feel again so you know what fills you up emotionally.

What do you want to be known for at the end of your life? Here are some examples from my life:

- Being a guide who inspires people to be their best self
- Being a leader who challenges people to achieve more than they ever thought possible

12

- Having a mind that dreams bigger than people think is realistic
- Being one who creates an environment where people feel respected and loved
- Being the individual who always believes "where there is a will, there is a way"

# PURPOSE FORMULA: VALUES + STRENGTHS + PASSIONS = PURPOSE

Write down things you value and then write down the strengths they coincide with. The things you value bring you the greatest joy, which gives you passion and purpose. My values are listed as an example:

| VALUES | STRENGTHS |
|---|---|
| Being present and connected with myself, my children, and grandchildren | Love |
| Having meaningful relationships and a deep connection to people | Loyal |
| Guiding and empowering others through my work | Intuitive |
| Enjoying nature and the beauty in the world | Spiritual |
| Leading a balanced life with great nutrition, and doing yoga every day | Health Consciousness |
| Being financially independent and only working because I love it | Passion |
| Living life fully and courageously every day of my life | Courage |

I suggest that you weed out the things in your life that are no longer serving you and are keeping you from doing the things in life you love. Prioritize the things in your list so that you nurture them on a daily basis.

# DEFINE WHO YOU WANT TO BE

Being *on purpose* means living your life intentionally, with purpose to all your actions. The meaning and purpose of your life is for you to become the best person you can be. When you discover yourself and define who that best person is that you want to become, everything begins to make sense. Until you discover your essential purpose, little else makes sense.

*"Don't be afraid your life will end; be afraid that it will never begin."*

—Grace Hansen

What are the things you want in life? Do you seek the things that money can buy or the things that money cannot buy? If you had to rank the following in order, how would you rank them?

- Possessions
- Personal relationships
- Professional success

People today are more distracted and busier than at any point in history. Many people have lots of material possessions and are highly interconnected through their social activities, but still something is missing for most people. Many people perceive their life purposes in relation to success in the workplace and financial independence. For example, many people allow themselves to be part of a culture of people who rush around and work too much so that they can indulge themselves in material possessions.

Most people want to put (or say that we do put) personal relationships first, but in what way? Do you spend time with your friends and loved ones in deep, intimate conversation about yourself, your relationships, your purpose, and how to live out your days with intention? Or, do you spend time with them running here and there—to the mall, to the movies, to the next commitment in a long list of commitments? Do you have real conversations, or do you have sound-bite conversations that may come close to intimacy—"sharing" about spouses, weight, a healthcare issue, or a family concern—but are lost as soon as there's an interruption?

Think about your life. Is it all caught up in rushing and consuming? What do you want it to be about? Can you visualize your life as you want it to be?

# SETTING GOALS

After discovering your purpose and what you want to achieve in the course of your life, you need to develop a goal. In order for something to be a goal, it must first be specific and measurable. Think of a goal as a dream with expectations. It is not a goal if you cannot define it fully or determine whether you achieve it.

Set goals that will stretch you to the limits without overwhelming you. This goal type is a "stretch goal." They must be sufficiently difficult, but not impossible. Remember that goal setting is important in developing your level of hope. Positive psychologists (Seligman, 2002) who study hope state that hope consists not only of willpower but also of meaningful goals to which one applies one's will.

*"If you do nothing unexpected, nothing unexpected happens."*

*—Fay Weldon*

Start by setting goals that will result in small victories that build your confidence in every area of your life. If you don't know what you want from life, everything will seem to be either an obstacle or a burden. By knowing what you want from life, you avoid the obstacle/burden struggle and doors of opportunity open for you and your wishes. One of the great lessons is that the whole world gets out of the way for people who know what they want or where they are going. Be assured; if you do not know where you are going, you are lost. You are never too young or too old to do what you want in life.

Tiger Woods was 3 years old when he shot 48 for nine holes on his hometown golf course. Mozart was 8 years old when he wrote his first symphony. Bill Gates was 19 years old when he cofounded Microsoft. Susan B. Anthony was 49 when she cofounded the National Woman Suffrage Association that eventually led to women's rights in the United States. Michelangelo was 72 when he designed the dome of St. Peter's Basilica in Rome. No matter your age, you can change your destiny.

There are moments when you might feel confused about your purpose in life. By living with the following core beliefs, your destiny will become much clearer:

- Believe that your attitudes and beliefs structure how the world appears and that your intuition is guiding you to fulfill your purpose.
- Honestly admit what is working in your life and what is not, and commit only to those things that have heart and meaning for you.
- Keep your life simple. You will attract people and events at the appropriate time, so let go of power and control.

Above all, remember that you always have a choice. The following are some suggestions that will help you stay focused on your purpose in all areas of your life:

- Control your physical cravings and do not be a slave to food, drink, or any other substance.
- Identify the people, activities, and possessions that are most important to you and give them your precious time.
- Cultivate the courage, determination, and persistence to choose the path that you are passionate about following and serve others in the process.
- Share your wealth with all you can. By doing so you will grow in personal wealth and never again be in need.
- Find true love with a soul mate who challenges and cherishes you.
- Maintain a sense of peace in knowing who you are.

# THE HAPPINESS PLAN

According to the National Academy of Sciences (Frederickson et al., 2013), happiness from having a purpose in life is linked with gene activity. Researchers found that inflammatory gene expression was low and antiviral and antibody gene expression was high among people who found joy from having a greater purpose in life. Conversely, people who found joy in just pleasing themselves had higher inflammatory gene expression and lower antiviral and antibody gene expression.

What this study tells us is that doing good and feeling good have very different effects on the human genome, even though they generate similar levels of positive emotion. Researcher Steven Cole, who is a professor of medicine at the University of California, Los Angeles, said in a statement, "Apparently, the human genome is much more sensitive to different ways of achieving happiness than are conscious minds" (Wheeler, 2013).

What is happiness? There are many definitions of the word *happiness* because it means different things to every person. Many people are often in search of happiness. One thing is certain, though; true happiness is joy that comes from within.

Do you have a plan to achieve and maintain happiness? In his best-selling book *The Four Agreements* (1997), Don Miguel Ruiz outlines a simple plan. His teachings have the basic premise that we create most of the drama and suffering in our lives and we block our own happiness, but we can choose to live another way. By refusing to buy into everything we've been taught about who we are, how the world works, and how we must react, and by making four simple pacts with ourselves, we can become dramatically happier regardless of our external circumstances. The following are the four agreements:

1. Be impeccable with your word—don't say it unless you mean it, and if there's gossip, don't repeat it.

2. Don't take anything personally—what other people say or do isn't about you; it's because of their own life experiences.

3. Don't make assumptions—preconceived ideas and rigid notions of how things should be lead to frustration and disappointment.

4. Always do your best—beating yourself up if you fail is pointless.

So many people prefer to live in drama because it's comfortable. For example, someone stays in a bad marriage or relationship because it's actually easier to stay where they know what to expect every day rather than leave and not know what to expect. They've practiced being the way they are for years and years, and they know exactly how to do it. They feel safe when they suffer. When they go into the unknown, they feel fear. Happiness is unknown. Love is unknown. To open the heart in trust is unknown. The old adage says love hurts, but it doesn't have to.

I can tell you that you really have only one mission in life, and that is to make yourself happy. The only way you can be happy is by being who you are. Living by these four principles will bring more joy into your being.

Being impeccable with your word applies not only to others but also to yourself because it will help you to live up to your values. Not taking anything personally does not mean that you will not have a reaction or you will not take action. We react in some way to most things in our lives, even those things that could potentially make us unhappy. When you take action you have clarity, you know exactly what you want, and you don't let emotions control you. The biggest assumption we make is that the story we've written about ourselves is true. We are the biggest mystery and the reason we are here is to know ourselves and be the best we can be.

In order to have complete peace and happiness, you have to surrender—it's like if you knew you were going to die, if you had only one day to live, you wouldn't care if you had money to buy things. You wouldn't care about anything except being happy. There's a kind of supreme trust that comes with surrendering.

People love because we have the capacity to love, and it feels good; it makes us happy. We feel like we have to justify love by being in a relationship, but that's not true. When someone says they love you, it's not about you; it's about them. Or if they hate you or they leave you, it's still not about you. The goal is to enjoy the life we have, which is a gift. The secret is for us to really enjoy life—and to be able to say to someone, "Hey, I love you." Who cares if they love you back?

Happiness is not dependent on a result, but on an action. That concept is really important. I think most people live their life for an end result, which is why they are never happy. A dancer is at his or her best when dancing, not when he or she is waiting for applause or accolades.

# 15 Questions to Find Alignment to Your Life Purpose

Take out a few sheets of loose paper and a pen. Find a place where you will not be interrupted. Answer each question with the first thing that pops into your head. Write quickly without editing. Give yourself less than 60 seconds to answer each question. Be honest.

1. What makes you smile? (List activities, people, events, hobbies, projects, and so on.)

2. What were your favorite things to do in the past? What about now?

3. What activities make you lose track of time?

4. What makes you feel great about yourself?

5. Who inspires you most? (This can be anyone you know or do not know: family, friends, authors, artists, leaders, and so on.) What qualities do those people have that inspire you?

6. What are you naturally good at? (Skills, abilities, talents)

7. What do people typically ask you for help with?

8. If you had to teach something, what would you teach?

9. What would you regret not fully doing, being, or having in your life?

10. Imagine you are 90 years old, sitting on a rocking chair on your porch. You can feel the spring breeze gently brushing against your face. You are blissful and happy, and you feel pleased with the won-

derful life you've been blessed with. Looking back at your life and all that you've achieved and acquired, all the relationships you've developed, what matters to you most? List them.

11. What are your deepest values? Use three to six words and prioritize the words in order of importance to you.

12. What were some challenges, difficulties, and hardships you've overcome or are in the process of overcoming? How did you do it?

13. What causes do you strongly believe in or connect with?

14. If you could get a message across to a large group of people, who would those people be? What would your message be?

15. Given your talents, passions, and values, how could you use these resources to serve, help, and contribute (to people, beings, causes, organizations, the environment, the planet, and so on)?

# ALIGNMENT WITH PURPOSE

In the 21st Century we are challenged with a new global economy and technology-driven world that is changing rapidly. Thomas Friedman (2005) calls it a "flat world" in that the playing field is level and individuals from around the planet can connect, communicate, and compete for our planet's limited resources. We are closing out the final chapters of the Industrial Age and opening up a new chapter that many believe is the "spiritual age." This spiritual age is not defined in a religious sense; it more broadly reflects the belief that the search for meaning and living a life of values and purpose is what is most important.

We can easily recognize those people, including ourselves, who are aligned with their purpose. The world is full of people who work too much, sleep too little, lead a sedentary lifestyle, eat food that lacks nutritional value, and never have enough time to spend with friends and family. It's time to refocus because that kind of lifestyle is destroying the well-being of many people.

Why is it so important to be aligned with your purpose? Because when you are *on purpose* you have more energy and true happiness in your life. Being in alignment with your purpose gives you peace. Peace is not the absence of pain. Peace is a certainty of living life for a worthy purpose, knowing that you are becoming a better person and touching the lives of others every day.

*"Life is not the way it's supposed to be. It's the way it is. The way you deal with it is what makes the difference."*

—Virginia Satir

## ARE YOU IN ALIGNMENT WITH YOUR PURPOSE?

There are many methods useful in identifying if you are in alignment with your purpose. For example, you may ask yourself, "Do I wake up most days feeling energized to go to work?" If the answer is "yes," then you may have an indication of your degree of alignment. Other questions to ask include, "Do my talents add real value to people's lives?" and "Can I be my authentic self at work?" At the end of the day, do you feel satisfied about how your day was spent? And when you are at home and with your family and friends, do you feel at peace and content?

It is important to align yourself with your purpose by prioritizing what is important to you. If you fail to do this, you are sacrificing your holistic health—physically, emotionally, intellectually, and spiritually. You must decide what is really important and necessary and make time for it. Otherwise, life keeps you distracted from what is really important. When you are attentive to your legitimate needs, you will find peace and fulfillment.

Your life is a vast array of choices that can bring you closer to the person you want to become. Bring into your life whatever you desire by deciding who you are and what you need to be happy. As Henry David Thoreau said, "If one advances confidently in the direction of one's dreams, and endeavors to live the life which one has imagined, one will meet with a success unexpected in common hours." Are you pursuing your dreams?

Balancing Act

# CREATING AN ELEVATOR SPEECH AND MISSION STATEMENT

Here is an exercise to help define your purpose. It sounds simple, but it is a very challenging exercise. Develop an "elevator pitch." Identify your life's purpose and learn to state it conversationally. If you can state your life's purpose to another person in the time it takes to ride an elevator—approximately 60 seconds—then you have clarity around your life purpose. Your elevator speech can become even more concise by making it into a mission statement. For example, my mission statement is, "Love, empower, motivate, and inspire others to live happier, healthier lives."

# SETTING GOALS

Create a goal that is SMART:

- **S**pecific
- **M**easureable
- **A**chievable
- **R**ealistic
- **T**imely

Example: You never eat vegetables but want to start. Don't expect to go from none to five a day. Instead, create a more realistic goal such as, "Beginning on Monday, I'll eat two servings of vegetables each day. I'll keep track of when I eat a vegetable by marking it on the calendar."

After you've eaten two servings of vegetables a day for some period of time (say, the next 3 weeks) then revise your goal upward to three servings of vegetables, and so on.

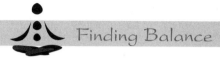

## Finding Balance

## REFLECTIONS

One's life has meaning. Ask yourself:

- Do I have a sense of purpose?
- Do I trust my intuition?
- Do I follow the happiness plan?
- Am I living my life with intention by fulfilling my bucket list?
- Who are the influential people in my life? What are their qualities?

## REFERENCES

Alderfer, C. (1972). *Existence, relatedness, and growth: Human needs in organizational settings.* New York: Free Press.

Carlson, E. (2013). Know thyself: How mindfulness can improve self-knowledge. *Perspectives on Psychological Science.* Association for Psychological Science, Washington, D.C. http://www.psychologicalscience.org/index.php/news/releases/know-thyself-how-mindfulness-can-improve-self-knowledge.html

Frankl, V. (1977). *Man's search for meaning.* New York: Pocket Books.

Fredrickson, B. L., Grewen, K. M., Coffey, K. A., Algoe, S. B., Firestine, A. M., Arevalo, J. M.,...Cole, S. W. (2013). A functional genomic perspective on human well-being. *Proceedings of the National Academy of Sciences, 110*(33), 13684-13689.

Friedman, T. (2005). *The world is flat: A brief history of the twenty-first century.* New York: Farrar, Straus and Giroux.

Maslow, A. H. (1943). A theory of human motivation. *Psychological Review, 50*(4), 370-396

Ruiz, D. M. (1997). *The four agreements: A practical guide to personal freedom.* San Rafael, California: Amber-Allen Publishing.

Seligman, M. E. P. (2002). *Authentic happiness: Using the new positive psychology to realize your potential for lasting fulfillment.* New York, NY: Free Press.

Wheeler, M. (2013). Be happy: Your genes may thank you. *UCLA Newsroom.* Retrieved from http://newsroom.ucla.edu/portal/ucla/don-t-worry-be-happy-247644.aspx

Zadan, C. (Producer), Meron, N. (Producer), & Reiner, R. (Director). (2007). *The bucket list* [Motion picture]. USA: Warner Brothers.

"Life is really simple, but we insist on making it complicated."

—Confucius

# 2

# SIMPLIFY YOUR LIFE

*—Sharon M. Weinstein, MS, RN, CRNI, FACW, FAAN*

Maintaining a work/life balance is essential for our well-being. The best way to begin working toward that balance is to simplify your life. Keeping it simple is a voluntary process, and you have the power to achieve this goal. And, remember that you are not alone!

The health professions, like many others, are demanding and time consuming, and they require a commitment that often extends beyond the 40-hour workweek. Today, people work longer hours, have kids involved in more activities than ever before, and maintain a busier lifestyle. Sometimes, they are caught in the "sandwich generation"—that group of "boomers" with aging parents and kids at home!

Each of us, at one time or another, has felt overwhelmed. We hesitate to take a holiday because when we return, the paperwork will be piled sky-high. We hesitate to attend a professional development program for fear of the overwhelming volume of work that awaits our return. This chapter looks at how we can combat that overwhelmed feeling by identifying our challenges, simplifying our lives, and enjoying newfound balance.

# COMPLEXITIES OF LIFE

The sheer complexity of our lives creates internal distress and can wreak havoc on our bodies. Distress is a contributor to disease, often referred to as "dis-ease," or a disorder within the cells. There are trillions of cells in the human body, and we don't always treat them well. We drive ourselves sick from doing too much and then wasting time recovering and getting back into the swing of things. The cardiac system is overstimulated, the immune system is suppressed, and our hormones are out of balance. The complex endocrine system controls the way we respond to our surroundings and provides the proper amount of energy our bodies need to function. Hormone imbalances result in a multitude of diseases, including, but not limited to, diabetes, osteoporosis, pituitary disorders, thyroid conditions, and more. Although some are more serious than others, these conditions have debilitating effects on physical and emotional health and quality of life for increasing numbers of professionals, young and old. Davidson and colleagues (2003) remind us that mindfulness meditation can impact changes in our systems and in immune response.

*"I think people want very much to simplify their lives enough so that they can control the things that make it possible to sleep at night."*

—Twyla Tharp

Are there really only 24 hours in each day? Do we still calculate time the same way? Have technologies simplified or complicated our lives? Time has never slowed down nor has it sped up; people do. We are the answer to the problem of time; if we want more time, we need to look at ourselves and the way in which we live.

Procrastination is abundant, and complexity is addictive; we cannot always find a way out. I know, because I've been there. When I was first introduced to the concept of work/life balance in 2002, I realized that I needed to radically change my own life. I understood that simplification could have a very positive effect on my work, my family, and my health, and I set out on a mission to simplify my own life. For me, this required a huge paradigm shift, and likely will for you, too.

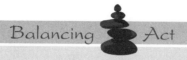

Balancing Act

# BEGINNINGS: YOUR TIME AND MINE

Have you ever thought that your life and your time were not your own? I have! And, it was true in so many ways. My life is simplified now, compared to the years between 1992 and 2004, when I worked about 100 hours per week and traveled monthly to countries in Eastern Europe. At that time, I directed the office of international affairs for a large hospital alliance, and 50% of my time was subcontracted to the United States Agency for International Development (USAID). My role was to foster international partnerships between U.S. hospitals and their foreign counterparts. I loved the work, I loved the people with whom I interacted, and I loved my job. The hours were extreme, and I found myself in a constant state of catching-up that left me always tired. Now, with a self-imposed work week of 40 hours, I feel I have dramatically simplified my life. I have time to work, write, teach, be with family, and give back to society. I have simplified my life by keeping up with less, not more.

I've taken lessons learned in less developed countries to heart as I have simplified my life. In my travels, I witnessed firsthand how simple life can be. Immediately following the earthquake in Yerevan, Armenia, on December 7, 1988, the only decent housing was in a former government hotel. Although the hotel offered neither heat nor hot water, I had a roof over my head and a clean bed. When there was no food in the hospital, our hosts found moldy bread. We ate this for weeks—sometimes with cheese or tomato sauce—and we always had an appreciation for what we had. Although it was impossible to get hot water in a tub, we could use an electric coil to warm some water and rinse the shampoo out of our hair. Our colleagues lacked so much, but their refinement of spirit and passion for their work were unsurpassed. They lived a simple life—nearly a sparse life—yet a life of gratitude.

Now, as I visit that same part of the world and see the progress that has been made, I am sometimes saddened by the fact that my colleagues are now living more complex lives, just as I once did. They too are burning the candle at both ends; they too are dealing with carpools, school-aged kids, aging parents, and work/life balance. Call it progress...I do not!

# YOUR COMMITMENTS

When you consider your commitments, your to-do or should-do list, do you procrastinate? Do you list the things that bring you greater pleasure at the top of the list, and the less desirable tasks at the bottom of that list (Fisher, 2011)? Simplifying one's life is a personal choice as well as a process. To start, examine your life and determine at least five areas that can be simplified (see the "Simplify by Five" sidebar later in this chapter). Although you may be habituated to taking care of all the laundry or dishes, can you release yourself from perfectionism and teach your kids or spouse how to do it? Even though it may take some restraint to keep from judging their efforts, identify the rewards for each of you if you successfully transition a task or responsibility to someone else in the household. What about the evening or morning routines, such as packing lunches or backpacks? Look closely at everything you do to identify five complicated parts of your life that can be simplified.

"Any intelligent fool can make things bigger, more complex, and more violent. It takes a touch of genius—and a lot of courage—to move in the opposite direction."

—E. F. Schumacker

I had the unfortunate experience of having a former home for sale for more than a year. Because of this, my family had to always be ready for an impromptu realtor visit with prospective buyers. Each and every day we had to make the beds, fill the dishwasher, put away the laundry, and clean the countertops. Because we had educated ourselves on all the "tips" for piquing a buyer's interest, we kept fresh flowers in the kitchen and bathrooms and maintained an uncluttered environment. We had to do all this while maintaining our already-complicated schedules. To help myself out, I had artificial floral arrangements created that mimicked fresh ones so that I could place them at a moment's notice. Although I would have preferred fresh flowers, I helped reduce the stress in my already stressful life by eliminating that small task.

With that 3,800-square-foot house sold, we planned to downsize. But we actually ended up with more room—5,200 square feet of space and much more than was needed for two people and a small dog. What were we thinking? What about simplicity? Was I complicating my life once again and creating more work, rather than less? Did creating more storage space mean that I could "collect" more stuff?

The new home was beautiful, and it represented our dream, which soon became our nightmare. Although new, and quite large, the home had structural challenges, local traffic challenges, and more. We realized our mistake, corrected the issues with a huge financial investment, and set out once again to sell not only the home but also 70% or more of the furnishings and fixtures. After all, if simplicity was our goal, we were going to get it right once and for all. The first step was to sell the property, and the second was to hire an estate sale professional, who ordered us out of the house while he and his team prepared for the sale, and processed potential buyers, payments, pickups, and more. What a simple process! I was finally getting it!

Currently we live an unencumbered life in a 2,000–square-foot town-home. We are not concerned with landscaping and snow removal. We travel if and when we choose to do so. We are free at last, and when we feel the need, we can pick up and move to a warmer location that is closer to those near and dear to us.

"Be content with what you have, rejoice in the way things are. When you realize there is nothing lacking, the whole world belongs to you."

—Lao Tzu

Balancing Act

## SIMPLIFY BY FIVE

Think of five areas in your life and begin your process to simplify. Write down each area. These areas could be work, food/nutrition, exercise, family, school, community, professional affiliations, and extracurricular activities.

## SOME SOLUTIONS

- Would your work go smoother if you spent a little time organizing before work? Look at everything you do on a daily basis and determine areas where you could be more efficient or can eliminate duplication. Propose changes to make yourself, your work, and your area more efficient. Hire a virtual assistant or college student to help with those things that consume your time and bring nominal rewards. Don't hesitate to "source" work out and to delegate to others. Assign it and trust that it will get done.

- Eat foods prepared simply, but eat with family and friends or make a ritual out of it, with each person being responsible for one aspect of the meal. Even school-age kids can be responsible for putting together a salad, fresh vegetable dish (or steamed vegetable with help from adults), and simple grains, and parents can trade off on the main course preparation. Everyone can work together before the beginning of the week to create a healthier menu and a meal plan, as well as do the shopping.

- Look at your community or professional affiliation responsibilities. Drop membership on a committee to free your time.

- Create a community with other parents to trade off carpooling to and from sports practice, drama club, scouts, the library, and so on. Stop driving all over town; consolidate your errands; order tickets and gifts online. Even groceries are available online and with delivery service.

- Clear out the clutter in your life to make it easier to find what you need. One solution is to process paperwork by handling it only once. Take action immediately on those items that require only a simple response. Create a system for managing follow-up items, whether a simple "tickler" file or by using a manual or electronic calendar. Consider a contact management system, sometimes referred to as CRM, so that your newsletters, appointments, and emails are done electronically. Put things in their place so that you can find them again.

- Do the laundry every other day and straighten up—but do not clean—every day.

- Turn on the TV only when you have a program to watch. Monitor media consumption and avoid disturbing news that brings you down. Record those shows that you would like to watch later.

Now that you are aware of the five simple steps, it is time to consider when enough is enough!

"It is the sweet, simple things of life which are the real ones after all."

—Laura Ingalls Wilder

# WHAT IS ENOUGH?

Everything in life is not black and white; there truly are shades of gray. Do you find yourself caught up in the good or bad, right or wrong, my-way-or-the-highway philosophy? It can be tempting to look at something with an all-or-nothing outlook. How do you know when to move on with your life, your job, your friends, and your relationship? People have the capacity to create things in our minds that do not really exist—that perhaps are untrue. How do you know what is authentic and what is not? How do you know when to stay and when to walk away? How do you avoid reading into something and making it a bigger deal than it really is? You need to know when enough is truly enough—and when it is time to move on.

There are three simple rules that can help you recognize and realize the consequences of "enough":

1. Trust actions rather than words.
2. Be as kind to yourself as you are to others.
3. Don't internalize blame—don't make it about you.

I am blessed that I discovered a simple ebook entitled *5 Elements of Success*. The author, Hui Chen (2011), shares his views on how you should be treated in life, and how you should treat others in return. Hui Chen speaks with a timeless wisdom that has enabled him to become a standard for *success through integrity*. He is one of the few Chinese billionaire entrepreneurs who is able to anticipate global trends that are decades ahead of their time.

He addresses the wisdom of ancient healing techniques based on the 5 Elements—Fire, Wood, Metal, Earth, and Water—and a belief system based on tradition, honor, excellence, vision, and humanity. The 5 Elements philosophy recognizes the strong interconnectedness present in all aspects of nature and the physical world. When I share this book with others, I refer to it as "life's little instruction manual." And, when I need to take action myself, I often think, "What would Hui Chen do or say?" I model my own behaviors by his thoughts and actions—and it has simplified my life and my responses. See Chapter 12 for more information on finding the 5 Elements within you.

Much like the philosophy of yin and yang states that all things in life are interconnected, so too are our bodies; if we wish to see targeted change, we must attend to the whole body. Well-being, vitality, stability, good health, and longevity can materialize only when all things—such as our vital organs and immune system—are in balance with one another. When we feel better, we live better. When we respect those around us, we reap the rewards of a life in balance.

# MINDLESS CONSUMPTION

*"We belabour, I think, under a very heavy crust of consumerism really."*

—Emma Thompson

Do you have too much "stuff"? Do you allow it to get the best of you? Are you overwhelmed? Mindless consumption allows stuff to overwhelm us. Most of us mindlessly consume stuff, wasting precious time in the process. For example, I have often thought that some children's playrooms resembled the LEGO Store. How many LEGOs could one possibly need? How can one, two, or three children possibly keep track of what goes where?

Regardless of our age, we are victims of consumerism. Consumerism is a social illness; we acquire no longer for survival but rather for mindless consumption. Then, why do we shop for what we do not need and perhaps cannot afford? Life is indeed good—we probably do not need more of the same thing, like LEGOs, if we already have enough. I recall that during one holiday season my grandson offered a list of what he would "like" to have and a list of what he "needed" to have. Why don't we, as adults, consider similar lists? Do we want a particular thing, or do we truly need it?

We are commodity-driven, and yet our most priceless commodity is our time. Time—especially time for ourselves—is truly what we need more of. Be intentional about you and your life. Be good to *you*. Set a time for yourself when you avoid mindless consumption each and every day. Make an actual date with yourself—for 30 minutes or more per day—when you turn off the TV, phone, computer, blog, or notepad. Close your eyes and relax. Regroup and revitalize *you*.

# Apps That Simply Life

We now ask, "Is there an app for that?" Imagine how things were several years ago and consider whether you would have asked that question, or whether you even knew what it meant. Career plus home plus family equates to a lot on your to-do list. How much time do you spend on Facebook, LinkedIn, Twitter, Pinterest, and other social sites per week, per day, or perhaps per hour? Is that wasted time that could be better spent on something else? Consider the suggestions in Chapter 6, but also consider using an application like Hootsuite that enables you to schedule your posts; create them in a single day, and schedule them for the week. This is simplicity! This is a digital detox. Ask yourself, "What makes the app work for me?" It must save time, be multiplatform or sync to multiple platforms, be used several times weekly, and improve your life.

## Apps That Simplify Your Day

- **Dropbox**—Use it to maintain your desktop, photos, and files. I use it as a backup (www.dropbox.com).

- **getAbstract**—Learn the key ideas in books within 10 minutes (www.getabstract.com).

- **Key Ring**—Manage rewards and loyalty cards (https://keyringapp.com).

- **ZipList**—Create shopping lists (http://get.ziplist.com).

- **RedLaser**—Scan barcodes and comparison-price shop (http://redlaser.com).

- **Evernote**—Manage electronic notes and paperwork (http://evernote.com/).

- **LastPass**—Consolidate your passwords (https://lastpass.com).

- **CalenGoo**—Sync your Google calendar across Android devices (http://android.calengoo.com).

- **Things 2**—Sync your Google calendar across Apple devices (http://culturedcode.com/things/iphone/?r-100).

- **Conciergist**—Talk or instant message (chat) with an agent who can answer questions or provide assistance (http://conciergist.com).

- **Any.do**—Stay organized with reminders and speech recognition (www.any.do/).

## Balancing Act

Think about your habits. We tend to love our habits; we are comfortable with the same old, same old—a routine that works. Think about the response you get when you ask a staff member why she does things the way she does. Perhaps the response is, "We've always done it that way." You can keep your habits, but change your choices.

Use the following questions to examine habits to try to understand the "why" behind them:

- Do habits evolve overnight, or are they long term? Why?

- Why do practically all dieters gain the weight back?

- We easily acquire bad habits, but what should we do to easily acquire good ones?

- Why are some people able to resist habit-forming behaviors?

- Why are one-third of Americans noncompliant with medication prescribed for a chronic illness?

- Do the same strategies that work for changing simple habits (tooth-flossing) also apply to complex habits (drinking less)?

- Why do we continue to consume what we know is not good for us—sugar, white flour, and more?

- What must we do to change our ways and make wiser choices?

*"Instead of wondering when your next vacation is, maybe you should set up a life you don't need to escape from."*

—Seth Godin

# Quantum Leaps

Personal growth is a challenge. When you experience a huge change in your life, it is a quantum leap (Wolf, 2010). It allows you to minimize, or to eliminate, some of the limiting beliefs that consume you, or that control your life and your actions. Personal growth often involves a shift in mind-set. I often thought that success takes hard work; if success came easily to me, I thought I must be doing something wrong. In retrospect, I realize that I worked hard for everything in my life. Nothing came that easily; rather, a shift in mind-set allowed me to achieve success and fostered my determination not to settle for less than the best.

Do you have limiting beliefs that consume you, or that control your life and your actions? Are you overdue for a shift in mindset? What might that look like?

What are you willing to settle for? Do you want a personal breakthrough or more of the same? You are working on simplifying and uncluttering. Prepare for a quantum leap. Timing is everything. Sometimes that quantum leap is in the area of personal and professional growth. It may be related to a sustained effort on your part. The following simple steps can facilitate the leap process:

- Totally immerse yourself in your goal or affirmation; write it down and repeat it daily.
- Know what it will take to achieve your goal; become an expert.
- Create the change by altering your own environment in support of your goal.

- Rethink and consider changing those with whom you spend your time. Why? Because they may cause you to question your abilities; they may stifle your growth; they may drain your energy. Surround yourself with those who bring you up, rather than those who drag you down.

Always think in the positive. For example, your affirmation might be, "I am so happy and proud now that I have reorganized my life and my time—now that I have taken the time to be with others, to share successes, and to create abundance in my life." When affirmations are done with intention and positive feelings, they transition you through the quantum leap.

## THE MAN WHO THINKS HE CAN

If you think you are beaten, you are;
If you think you dare not, you don't;
If you'd like to win, but think you can't,
It's almost a cinch you won't.
If you think you'll lose, you're lost,
For out in the world we find
Success begins with a fellow's will,
It's all in the state of mind.

If you think you're outcasted, you are;
You've got to think high to rise.
You've got to be sure of yourself before
You can ever win a prize.
Life's battles don't always go
To the stronger or faster man;
But soon or later the man who wins
Is the man who thinks he can.

This poem is attributed to Walter D. Wintle, who lived in the late 19th and early 20th centuries. The first known publication date of the poem is 1905. It was published in *Poems That Live Forever*, compiled by Hazel Felleman, 1965.

If you keep on doing what you have done in the past, chances are you will achieve the same results. If you try harder at doing the same thing, you may make an incremental gain, but not a quantum leap. More of the same is a trap. To truly switch gears, you need to recognize that what you do is more important than how you do it.

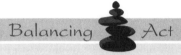

Balancing Act

### LIFE'S BALANCING ACT

You can create your own balancing act. Start by warming up. Balance on one foot and remain in that position for 2 minutes; think about what you are experiencing while you are "on hold." What did you notice, and what did you most want to do? Think about the changes in your environment that affect your own balancing act. If you are in a cold room, your body shivers. If you are in a warm room, your body sweats. This is a cause-and-effect reaction. Develop a cause-and-effect chart of your own and include those activities that are related to work and home. Then examine areas of imbalance and make steps to jumpstart your own life in balance.

It's in your power. Make a quantum leap and achieve a personal breakthrough!

# THE LAWS OF LIFE

Universal laws have emerged over time; they represent natural principles and outcomes in life, and are generally referred to as The Laws of Life. Over the years, many public figures have jumped on The Laws of Life bandwagon, including Dr. Phil, Tony Robbins, and others. Their interpretations vary from Dr. Phil's, "You either get it or you don't," to the more refined "Celebration of Spirit" from John Marks Templeton. Whereas Dr. Phil addresses life as we live it today, Templeton ponders what it means to live the good life.

I want to cover three of these Laws of Life in more detail to demonstrate how you can use them to simplify and decompress:

- The law of attraction
- The law of intention
- The law of abundance

*"Never interrupt someone doing something you said couldn't be done."*

*—Amelia Earhart*

## THE LAW OF ATTRACTION

The concept of the law of attraction is extremely simple: We attract whatever we choose to give our attention to—whether wanted or unwanted. It does not matter who you are, where you live, what your religious beliefs are, or in what year you were born. It is true for everyone equally. After you understand the law of attraction, there is no looking back. It will be part of you forever. Although promoted in *The Secret* by Rhonda Byrne, this law has been handed down through history. Great thinkers—Plato, Aristotle, Socrates, Michelangelo, Newton, Franklin, Jefferson, and many others—knew this tenet of life.

*"Everything you want is out there waiting for you to ask. Everything you want also wants you. But you have to take action to get it."*

*—Jack Canfield*

The simplest definition of this law is *like attracts like.* Other definitions include:

- You get what you think about.
- You think that things will be negative, and they will.
- You think that things will be positive, and they will.

- You are a living magnet.
- You get what you put your energy and focus on.
- Energy attracts like energy.

Experiment with it. If you normally think negatively, decide that you will spend one whole day thinking positively. Pay close attention and track the subtle and not-so-subtle differences in your new positive thoughts. Consider as you go along that you have a choice as to how to react to everything that happens to you.

*"The more clearly we can focus our attention on the wonders and realities of the universe about us, the less taste we shall have for destruction."*

*—Rachel Carson*

## THE LAW OF INTENTION

Intentions are much more powerful than wants, wishes, or hopes. Intention releases a force that makes things happen. If you intend for something to occur, it will because the force of the universe backs your vision. That is the power of intention—the power behind desire. Alone, intention may be strong and desire may be weak simply because you must be attached to the outcome (to your desire) to make it a reality.

Your intention is for the future, but your attention must be in the present in order for it to manifest itself. Karma is a reflection of our intentions. Karma is the intentional action that creates a result. When your intentions are grounded, they represent the highest good rather than your own ego. The ego makes us think, "What's in it for me?" We often think of karma in terms of good and bad. We refer to it as the energy in a room or the work environment. Wholesome karma is good karma, which produces acts that result in compassion, wisdom, and kindness.

*"All great acts are ruled by intention. What you mean is what you get."*

*—Brenna Yovanoff*

## The Law of Abundance

Abundance is so much more than financial gain; it relates to a connection to our source of energy. Abundance is ours; how we experience it varies according to our own alignment. We draw to ourselves any and all things that are in sync with our heart's energy. This includes health, wealth, joy, creativity, gratitude, and self-awareness. Three key factors effect abundance, and they include where we focus our attention, what we accept and believe we deserve, and our own experience or lack thereof in being open to and receiving it. Many of us have never been taught how to receive. In order to receive, we must let go of resistance and open ourselves to abundance.

*"Let a person radically alter his thoughts and he will be astonished at the rapid transformation it will effect in the material conditions of his life."*

*—James Allen*

## KEEPING LIFE SIMPLE

Life is actually pretty simple, but remember that simple does not mean easy. It does mean manageable. To truly simplify, you must know where you are, and where you want to be. You must recognize those things that overwhelm you, occupy perhaps too much time, and deplete your energy.

So, assess your current situation, and ask yourself why you do what you do and how you might be able to shift priorities to gain much-needed time, space, or resources. Examine how the laws apply to your own life.

For example, the Law of Attraction states that we attract into our lives what we project into the universe. Thus, using the tools in this chapter, if we assess and revise our projections, we can simply attract positive vibrations and energies that will lead to a life in balance. Don't be afraid to just be who you are and to do what you think is right. Don't be afraid to light up the world with your own intentions, your own energy, and your own simplicity. Live the good life (Templeton, 2012).

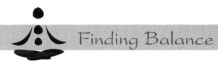

## Finding Balance

### YOUR SCORECARD

You can't walk the pathway to balance unless you understand where you currently stand. Complete the following survey to get an idea of where your strengths and weaknesses lie. Implement some of the ideas in this book, and then, a few months from now, retake the survey and see how you have improved.

### MY BALANCE SCORECARD

1. How would you describe your current weight?

    ____Normal    ____Overweight

2. How would you describe your current exercise level?

    ____Active    ____Inactive

3. If you do not exercise, what is your main reason?

    ____Time    ___Energy

4. How many hours of sleep did you get last night?

    ____Less than 6    ____More than 7

5. How many 8-ounce glasses of water do you drink a day?

    ___Less than 8    ____More than 8

6. Do you have problems with focus?

    ___Yes    ___No

7.  Describe your current energy level.

    ___High   ___Low

8.  How would you describe your motivation to eat healthy?

    ____Good   ___Poor

9.  How would you describe your morale?

    ___Good   ___Poor

10. What factor plays the greatest part in your overall health?

    ___Self-motivation

    ___Employer support

    ___Time

    ___Money

11. Are you a "collector" of things/stuff/items that you do not necessarily need?

    ___Yes   ___No

12. Do you powernap to relieve stress?

    ___Yes   ___No

Date _____

# REFLECTIONS

- Reflect on your own life and celebrate the goodness within.
- Accept transformation and the need for change.
- Know when enough is enough.
- Think abundance, and act intentionally.

# References

Chen, H. (2011). *5 elements of success*. Richmond, BC: Alphay. Retrieved from http://www.alphayglobal.com/portals/0/pdf/five_elements_of_success.pdf

Davidson, R. J., Kabat-Zinn, J., Schumacher, J., Rosenkranz, M., Muller, D., Santorielli, S. F.,…Sheridan, J. F. (2003). Alterations in brain and immune function produced by mindfulness meditation. *Psychosomatic Medicine, 65*(4), 564-570.

Fisher, L. (2011). The power of procrastination: How can we use procrastination creatively? *Untangling Life's Complexities*. [Web log post]. Retrieved from http://www.psychologytoday.com/blog/untangling-lifes-complexities/201111/the-power-procrastination

Templeton, J. M. (2012). *The essential worldwide laws of life*. West Conshohocken, Pennsylvania: Templeton.

Wolf, F. (2010). *Taking the quantum leap: The new physics for nonscientists*. New York: Harper Collins.

*"Reality is the leading cause of stress among those in touch with it."*

*—Lily Tomlin*

# 3

# THE WAGES OF STRESS

*—Sharon M. Weinstein, MS, RN, CRNI, FACW, FAAN*

We hear about stress every day. It affects both the mind and the body. Job stress increases the risk of cardiovascular disease and the development of back- and upper-extremity musculoskeletal disorders. The differences in rates of mental health problems, such as depression and burnout, for different occupations may be partly due to differences in job stress level. Clearly, people can reap significant benefits from reducing the stress in their lives at work and home.

But before you can create a formula for stress relief, you need to better understand the complex phenomena causing your heart to be over-stimulated, your immune system to be suppressed, your hormonal output to be unbalanced, and your reproductive system to function abnormally. This chapter explores stress, what we need to know, and how that knowledge can help to reduce it.

# What Is This Thing Called Stress?

The physiology of stress can be described as a specific response by the body to a stimulus, such as pain or fear, that disturbs or interferes with the normal physiological equilibrium of an organism.

*"It's better to oversleep and miss the boat than get up early and sink."*

—Elizabeth Jane Howard

Stress is not unusual or abnormal. It's an everyday response by the body to an event. Your heart rate and respiration increase in anticipation of muscular activity. Stress is what your body experiences as it adjusts to ever-changing circumstances.

As a positive influence, stress can fill you with excitement and propel you into action or provide you with a feeling of happiness. Stress can be very motivating. It enables you to accomplish tasks and set goals and see them through to completion. This "good" stress is associated with the release of adrenaline, endorphins, serotonin, and dopamine, all of which act as natural antidepressants and pain relievers in the body.

The body is amazing: It pumps adrenaline through your system in response to stress, but if you do not use up the adrenaline, it will manifest itself negatively in stress-induced tension, muscle pain, and more. Thus, a natural cycle within our bodies both relieves and contributes to stress.

# Sources of Stress

In today's economic environment, stress may be attributed to having a job, as much as to not having one. There are massive layoffs around the country, and they impact workers in all settings, including healthcare. If an employee fears the loss of a job, even a job that is not the best, he or she is stressed. How will the family be fed? How will they pay their bills?

Will they have to think twice before making routine purchases? People have different stress triggers, but work tops the list.

## CAUSES OF WORK-RELATED STRESS

Being unhappy in your job

A heavy workload or too much responsibility

Working long hours

Poor management, unclear expectations of your work

Lack of input in the decision-making process

Working under dangerous conditions

Being insecure about your chance for advancement or risk of termination

Bullying

# DISTRESS OR EUSTRESS

When the body is acidic, there is distress at the cellular level. Stress has become uncontrollable, prolonged, or overwhelmingly destructive. Stress contributes to chronic disease, and you need to eliminate the stressors in your environment that affect your ability to be balanced. In general, we associate distress with "bad" stress—the stress that takes a physical toll on the body. "Positive" stress, called *eustress*, evolves from the anticipation of joy, a new birth, physical exercise, graduation, and/or excitement. Although the symptoms of the two types of stress may be similar, eustress can create a good feeling as your body releases endorphins. It motivates you to continue down that ski slope or to the finish line of a half marathon.

# SYMPTOMS

If you are suffering from some of the following symptoms, it may indicate that you are feeling the effects of stress. If you find that work or aspects of your work bring on or make these symptoms worse, speak to your manager, trade union representative, or your human resources/talent management department. Sometimes an early intervention can alleviate the symptoms.

| Emotional Symptoms | Mental Symptoms | Other Symptoms |
| --- | --- | --- |
| Depression or sadness | Confusion, indecision | Changes in eating habits |
| Disappointment with self | Inability to concentrate | Sleep disturbances |
| Easily upset and tearful | Memory changes unrelated to aging, physical illness, or medication | Gastric problems |
| Feeling lonely, withdrawn | | Headaches |
| Lack of motivation | | Increased use of substances such as tobacco and alcohol |
| Mood swings | | |

# Adaptagenicity

It is impossible to address stress without including adaptagenicity. Adaptagenicity is the body's ability to deal with stress, and everyone needs it. You are familiar with antioxidants—nearly every media advertisement speaks to the need for antioxidants. Chen, Liou, and Chang (2008) studied the direct relationship between the antioxidant potential of three adaptogen extracts. They concluded that the supplementation of adaptogen extracts containing high levels of polyphenols may not only have adaptogen properties, but may decrease the risk of complications caused by oxidative stress.

What happens when a body is out of balance? When a body is out of balance, unpaired electrons, or "free radicals," cause damage and stress to cells and tissues; the process is known as *oxidation*. You may be familiar with oxidative stress if you reside near a beach or ocean and park your bicycle or vehicle in close proximity to sea water. The rust that develops on the vehicle is oxidative stress. Oxidative stress plays a significant role in many human diseases, including heart disease, diabetes, and cancer (Chen et al., 2008).

But, have you heard of polysaccharides? Polysaccharides are super antioxidants that strengthen the cells. They adapt to different viruses. They activate important immune supporters such as Natural Killer and T cells, which are particularly important in preventing tumor growth and cancer viruses from invading healthy cells (Baltra, Sharma, & Khajuria, 2013). And polysaccharides are readily found in edible and medicinal mushrooms. The mushroom industry is growing exponentially, and there are more than 1,300 edible varieties and 700 medicinal forms. They have been used in Eastern medicine for years, and they are now accepted in the West. Let me be clear, these are not the "shrooms" that you may have taken in school. We are not talking about lava lamps, tie-dye, and more. We are talking about research in progress at Johns Hopkins Medical Center, the University of Minnesota, and other research facilities. Jiang and Sliva found that a mushroom blend including Ganoderma lucidum could suppress growth and invasiveness of human breast cancer cells (2010).

Mushrooms can be used every day as part of a healthy diet, and the great thing is they are a "whole food," not a supplement or a medicine. You do not need to be a clinician to decide how to use them. You can take them in capsules or in coffee. Try opening the capsules, adding the powder to a recipe, a smoothie, or cup of tea. Hippocrates said, "Let food be your medicine." He may have been correct!

Medicinal mushrooms are adaptogenic (stress-reducing), functional foods that stimulate different systems of your body. Adaptogenic, functional foods work together to create synergism in the body. This brings balance and health. Unlike a drug, they become part of your cell structure and work over time. Adaptogens help eliminate toxins, strengthen the immune system, and have a balancing effect without harmful side effects. For example, if you have high blood pressure, an adaptogen targets weak cells in the circulatory system to provide balance, thereby strengthening the cells and their functions (Preuss, Echard, Bagchi, & Perricone, 2010).

# STRESS AND CHOLESTEROL LEVELS

A negative reaction to stress can be reflected in cholesterol levels. Steptoe and Marmot (2003) have consistently researched population groups, work roles, and more to identify factors affecting both cholesterol and blood pressure levels. Stress may raise cholesterol levels, both immediately and over the long term and those who reacted more strongly to emotional situations also demonstrated immediate and significant increases in cholesterol level. In a subsequent study, these same study participants who initially responded more dramatically to stressful situations experienced a more significant elevation in cholesterol levels than other study participants. How significant? Those who had initial stress responses in the top third of the group were more likely to have readings above the recommended levels for cholesterol than participants whose initial stress responses fell in the bottom third (Brydon & Steptoe, 2005).

So, what is the stress-cholesterol connection? Although researchers aren't certain, one theory is that stress might increase the body's inflammatory processes, which, in turn, increases lipid production.

# WORKPLACE STRESS

Longer hours, greater workloads, staff reductions: These and other factors contribute to stress in the workplace. A healthy workplace helps combat stress. For those who work shift work, stress is a constant. Shift work disorder (SWD) is a circadian rhythm disorder (see Chapter 9). About 20% of the workforce in the United States is involved in rotating shifts;

their schedules are in direct conflict with the body's normal rhythm (Kolla & Auger, 2011). These workers experience difficulty adjusting to their diverse sleep and wake schedules. The consequences may be extreme and contribute to increased accidents, sick leave, irritability, and even work-related errors. It is also a form of stress.

Stress affects fatigue, safety, retention, and outcomes. Healthcare leaders have been challenged by the American Association of Critical-Care Nurses (AACN), other professional organizations, and regulatory agencies to develop and sustain healthy work environments that support the professional practice of nursing. Magnet designation, the Beacon award, and other organizational structures and cultures led by authentic and transformational leaders have been the stimulus to ensure that workplaces are healthy and healthful.

According to the Towers Watson 2011/2012 survey, there is a strong link between highly effective health and productivity strategies and strong human capital and financial results. The study further reports a savings in annual health care costs per employee of $1000. This gives a company with 10,000 employees a $10 million cost advantage. Achievement of healthy work environments requires transformational change, with interventions that target underlying workplace and organizational factors. The trend toward healing environments within the workplace is aimed at overall well-being.

# HEALING WORK ENVIRONMENTS

Workplace health and wellness initiatives have positive implications for both organizations and staff. Studies have found that implementation of wellness programs can result in better health for employees and lower healthcare costs for organizations.

A simple example of a wellness initiative is offering chair massage at little or no charge to employees. My former employer offered it on a monthly basis, and there was always a waiting list for this amazing stress-reducing treatment.

Features associated with a healing environment might be structural or more ambient, such as controlled lighting, sharing circles, and waterfalls. Florence Nightingale's theory of nursing is a reminder that nursing is a calling. Her vision honored the relationship between the patient and the nurse and called for an awareness of the environment. A caring environment that acknowledges the mind/body/spirit connection is invaluable to nurses as well as to patients. The environment is realized through respect, support, and open communication, which creates a culture of magnetism. Taking a holistic approach encourages healing in all dimensions—mental, emotional, spiritual, social, and physical—thus creating an optimal environment of renewal for all—a Circle of Wellness.

Wellness is about taking responsibility, being accountable, and living consciously. Wellness is a choice—a decision to move toward optimum health and a lifestyle you design to achieve your highest potential for well-being. Trust your body and your soul. Everyone is unique, and wellness is thus different for each of us. It is essential that each person learn to read and interpret the internal and external signals that your body is giving you all the time about what you need and want for balance, healing, and greater vitality. Nurses can easily do this!

My practice interest is in offering solutions for health, wellness, safety, and the environment. I collaborate with organizations that insure between 5 and 5,000 lives, and I help them to maintain healthcare costs through WorkingWell programs (http://smwgroupllc.com). I also work with entrepreneurs, helping them to envision the next phase of their nursing careers and executing the process.

So, regardless of the work that you do or the skill sets that you bring to the table, step back, look at the big picture, and use that perspective to help people feel good about themselves. That is the critical skill that's enabled me to touch the lives of people like you and me on a global scale! I can combine my background in western medicine with integrative and functional medicine to help people feel better and live longer naturally. From experience, I know that sometimes success comes down to the environment in which we live and work. That environment can hinder our ability to be well and can create stress-induced illness. This can take a huge toll on energy levels and the feeling of well-being we all rely on to have optimal vitality and wellness.

*"Men, for the sake of getting a living, forget to live."*
—Margaret Fuller

# THE WAGES OF STRESS: COST FACTORS

*Workplace wellness* is a holistic concept that touches on many aspects of an organization and how it is managed. Successful workplace health and well-being programs are supported by senior management and form an integral part of the organization's strategy. Comprehensive workplace wellness plans typically comprise a range of programs and activities related to physical environment, health practices, and social environment.

Stress-induced symptoms account for nearly 90% of physician-office visits (WebMD, 2014). If we could eliminate some of the stressors, and thus the symptoms, we might minimize cost factors. Clearly, a work environment that includes insults, backstabbing, and belittling can erode an employee's morale. What's less understood is that such a toxic work atmosphere can also lead to deteriorating health.

## THE COST TO FAMILY

I recall a time when my adult children said that they were not going to be calling me anymore. They preferred to speak to their dad, who paid attention to the conversation. At the end of a call they would test me on what they had said, and although I could repeat, nearly word for word, their comments, my background typing and shuffling of papers made me pay a price! Family is important, and family time should be just that—family time. Put away the cellular device and pay attention; doing so will minimize stress for you and the family as a whole.

## The Cost of Conflict and Confrontation

Difficult people generate difficult work settings; a workplace may seem like a battlefield with a conflict at every turn in the road or within each department. Conflict is inevitable, and experiencing some conflict at work does not mean that it is time to seek another job. Instead, remember that it takes two to tango. Take ownership for your part in the disagreement so that you may move on. Allow yourself time to cool off before addressing the issue and apologizing as appropriate. Time does heal wounds as you both move ahead.

For example, I recall a time at a prominent medical school in the Chicago area when one of the clinical chairs was a source of constant conflict for me. I found it beneficial to type a response, print it out, lock it in my drawer, and shred it the following morning. My assistant found it beneficial to hang a soft dartboard behind her door. In the center, she placed a headshot of the offender. She actually threw darts, removing them before leaving her office. It was extreme, but it gave her great relief from an otherwise confrontational situation.

## The Cost to Relationships

The American Institute of Stress (n.d.) identifies four main causes of workplace anxiety: workload (46%), conflicts with other people (28%), juggling personal and professional time (20%), and lack of job security (6%). Managing stress is everyone's job. Owners and managers can be transparent, avoid overloading staff, ask for input, and cultivate a positive work setting. Staff can recognize possible warning signs, take care of their bodies, manage their time wisely, and simplify (see Chapter 2).

## The Cost to Health

Stress may very well be the health epidemic of the 21$^{st}$ century. According to the American Psychological Society (2012), stress costs U.S. businesses roughly $300 billion a year as a result of absenteeism, reduced productivity levels, and employee turnover. Companies are also paying higher medical and insurance fees. For example, the National Institute for

Occupational Safety and Health (n.d.) reports that job stress prompts longer periods of employee disability than other types of work-related injuries or illnesses do. In general, employers want employees to be happier and healthier every day. Regardless of the setting—corporate, social, or home life—we all want to live a healthier, happier life.

Employee emotional, physical, and mental health are huge issues. Procrastination and missed deadlines, difficulties with memory and listening, morale, and withdrawal are all warning signs of an overstressed employee. The stigma associated with depression, however, still remains. Employee Assistance Programs (EAPs) have been assets to employers and their staffs for many years.

My nephew, a partner at a prominent law firm, committed suicide after years of depression. His spouse has worked diligently to have legislation passed in her state that mandates healthcare professionals' preparedness in the screening, assessment, and treatment of those who are suicidal. The Matt Adler Suicide Assessment, Treatment & Management Act was signed into law in 2012. It requires that mental health professionals licensed in the state of Washington, at least once every 6 years, complete a training program of 6 hours or longer in suicide assessment, treatment, and management that is approved by the relevant disciplining authority. The goal is to enhance awareness of depression, and to be proactive in addressing it, rather than reactive (Stuber, 2012).

From a physical perspective, we all know employees who show up sick; perhaps they fear losing income or employment if they call in sick. The result is *presenteeism*—being physically at work without being totally engaged. A systematic process that screens all employees for contagious illnesses at the start of their shifts may limit the impact of presenteeism (see Chapter 5). Stephens (2013) addresses the implications and health risks of presenteeism as a productivity drain and its real cost to employers.

## HEALTHCARE COSTS

As stated previously, presenteeism occurs when an employee goes to work despite a medical illness that will prevent him or her from fully functioning at work. This problem has been well studied in the business and social science literature (Widera, Chang, & Chen, 2010) and carries increased importance in the healthcare setting due to the risk of infectious disease transmission in vulnerable patient populations. The costs associated with absenteeism are obvious, but presenteeism also takes a financial toll when others have to cover for the employee who is there, but not present.

## THE COST TO PERFORMANCE

Chronic health conditions, such as allergies, arthritis, depression, and diabetes, can result in significant productivity issues. And I've already noted previously how acute infectious illnesses pose an additional risk from presenteeism as employees can serve as a vector of disease transmission (Hansen & Andersen, 2008). Essentially, a person at work, but out of it and merely taking up space, may be out of it because of illness or because of a non-health related issue. However, no matter the cause, the result is often the same. That sort of presenteeism leads to productivity and performance issues, including safety concerns, equipment breakage or possible contamination (Fenelon, Holcroft, & Waters, 2009) and work-related accidents. A comprehensive workplace wellness program may be beneficial for employee health and the company's financial well-being. What drives healthcare workers to come to work while ill? The answer to this question is complex and it may depend on the job itself, the discipline of the employee, rank within the institution or organization, financial security, and the level of work involved.

# COPING

There are multiple ways in which you can make yourself more stress resistant. Coping mechanisms include stopping yourself from having guilty feelings, being decisive, and avoiding trying to be a perfectionist. Take good care of your emotional and physical self. Eat healthy, well-balanced meals, and exercise on a regular basis. Remember to give yourself a break—you deserve it!

# STRESS REDUCTION

Work isn't the only source of stress; home life can be just as hectic as work life. You need to reduce and manage stress both at work and at home. The body and mind need more short periods of rest than most people allow. Just a few minutes of total relaxation will refresh you so you can more effectively complete the task at hand. And, yes, you can learn to fully relax for a few minutes a day in your home or even in your office setting.

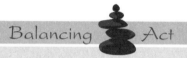

Balancing Act

## A SEASONAL EXPERIENCE IN THE FOREST

And, along comes forest bathing—the ideal walk in the woods—and it works any time of the year. To make it work, you must get started, especially when the days are longer and you are spending more time outside than at other times of the year. For many of us, the economy has limited the kinds of activities that we can do solo or as a family or group. Think about it—in the spring and summer, during allergy season, spending more time in nature could have surprising health benefits. In the fall, you get a double bonus; a walk in the woods provides fresh air and a sense of peace, and it also exposes you to the colorful array of leaves and nature. In the winter, the ground is covered with frost or snow, yet the air that you breathe is clean, cool, and invigorating. In a series of studies, scientists found that when people swap their concrete walls for some time with Mother Nature—forests, parks, and other places with plenty of trees—they experience increased immune function (Phillips, 2011).

The entire family can benefit from a walk in the woods. The kids will breathe good air, enjoy the benefits of nature, collect leaves, and scrapbook them when they get home. Parents will enjoy being outside with those nearest and dearest to them. They will enjoy nature through the eyes and ears of a child.

I had the privilege of working in Russia for nearly 10 years in the healthcare sector, and while I stayed in the city and used public transportation, I often thought about getting out of town for the weekend and enjoying the natural beauties of the country. My colleagues made it a point to visit their country homes on the weekends—even in the winter—to sit by a fire while inside, but also to experience nature in the forest outside. I had the joy of joining them on many occasions so that I could walk through the forest and revisit nature. What a difference it made in my own life! I was working 100-hour weeks, often traveling between cities and between countries in a week's time. I needed to relax, and I did not always make the time to do so. My "forest bathing" experience restored my own well-being and taught me an important lesson about self-care. You cannot care for others until you take care of yourself!

"Don't underestimate the value of Doing Nothing, of just going along, listening to all the things you can't hear, and not bothering."

—Pooh's Little Instruction Book, inspired by A.A. Milne

One strategy you can use is the power nap. In a study of 23,681 participants who were free of coronary heart disease, stroke, or cancer at the time of enrollment, researchers found that a regular nap reduced coronary mortality. For example, those who napped on a regular basis (at least three times a week for an average of at least 30 minutes) had a 37% lower coronary mortality compared to those who did not rest. Working men had the highest benefit (Naska, Oikoniomou, Trichopoulou, Psaltopoulou, & Trichopoulos, 2007).

A power nap will put you into a refreshing phase of sleep, but it's not so deep that you wake up feeling even more tired than before. A power nap should last from a few minutes up to a maximum of 20 minutes and can be done anywhere that's safe and appropriate.

"Sometimes the most important thing in a whole day is the rest we take between two deep breaths."

—Etty Hillesum

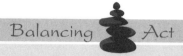
Balancing Act

Life really is a balancing act. Take a moment to think about your to-do list and the challenges of juggling work and play; friends and family; body, mind, and spirit; to achieve balance in your own life. The ability to find balance is a struggle and a journey, and stress is a common denominator that often gets in the way. In order to achieve balance, you must reduce stress. This sidebar discusses how!

*"So be sure when you step, Step with care and great tact. And remember that life's A Great Balancing Act. And will you succeed? Yes! You will, indeed! (98 and ¾ percent guaranteed) Kid, you'll move mountains."*

–Dr. Seuss

## STRESS-REDUCING TIPS

While you may not be able to fully relieve stress, you can learn to manage it. The first step is to realize that there are some things in your home lives and at work that you cannot control, but stress management begins and ends with you. By following these simple tips, you will be well on the way toward a stress-reduction pathway.

## BREATHING

Controlled breathing is a stress-relief technique that's fast, simple, and free. It can be done anywhere and at any time. It has numerous positive effects on your health, such as reducing high blood pressure. Controlled breathing, in storybook form, even works for stressed kids who need to relax before going to bed.

Here's how basic controlled breathing works:

- Sit or stand in a relaxed position.

- Slowly inhale through your nose. Fill your lungs with fresh air and let your abdomen expand outward, rather than raising your shoulders.

- Exhale slowly through your mouth. Pay attention to the exhale. Drag it out for as long as possible.

- Repeat this exercise over 2 or 3 minutes and feel the tension release from your body.

# EXERCISE

The human body needs to exercise to function properly. Exercise helps you think with more clarity, gives you more energy, and helps prevent diseases such as stroke and type 2 diabetes (Sarnataro, 2008).

# STRETCHING

It's a good idea to stretch before starting an exercise activity. If you have ever taken group or individual exercise classes, chances are that the trainer suggested stretching out before and after the activity. You see this action in household pets all of the time; they awaken and stretch their bodies before starting their days.

# SIMPLE EXERCISES

Walking is a very simple exercise and an excellent stress-relief technique. It doesn't require a lot of focus and can easily be incorporated into your workday, no matter how pressed for time you are. Take a brisk walk around the block, through your workplace, or up and down the stairs. Use up the adrenaline that's going through your bloodstream before it negatively affects your health.

# SLEEP

We now know the benefits of a power nap. A 15- to 30-minute nap in the afternoon increases alertness, improves cognitive functioning, and reduces stress (Scott, 2008).

Adequate nighttime sleep is also important. The body needs 8 hours per night, every night. The effects of lost sleep are cumulative and can result in impaired reaction time, vision, information processing, and short-term memory (Scott, 2008).

# EAT WELL

Eat well-balanced meals and take appropriate vitamins and minerals to make sure your body is adequately nourished and healthy. See Chapter 10 for more on a balanced life.

Maintain a healthy body fat-to-muscle ratio. If necessary, concentrate on losing fat instead of just losing weight. Skinny does not equal healthy. The starlets who influence teenagers are not role models for health. When one loses weight quickly, that weight is easily regained, plus some. Starvation causes muscle loss and can contribute to weakness and serious illness.

# POSTURE

Because adolescent girls hit their growth spurt earlier than boys, they sometimes slouch to avoid appearing taller. When I was a teenager, I remember parents reminding their daughters to sit upright, stand tall, and be proud of their height. The same adage continues to be true today. Remind yourself to maintain proper posture. If you sit most of the time, adjust the chair according to your body proportions. Keep your feet flat on the floor. Your rib cage should not rest on your hip joints.

Straighten your spine but don't hyperextend. Move your shoulders back, and take pressure off the spine in your neck by keeping your head aligned with the rest of the spine. I find that the use of a magnetized chair pad helps relieve pressure on the spine, and it improves my circulation at the same time.

# PRIORITIZE

Not everything needs to be taken care of *right now.* Recognize the difference between what is urgent and what is important, and manage your time wisely. Learn to say "no." Remind yourself that "no" is a complete sentence. Accept help when it's offered, or ask for help if you feel overwhelmed.

## SOLUTIONS

Stress management programs within the workplace and beyond are becoming more prominent. Drinking hot water with lemon has long been used by our Eastern colleagues as a stress remedy; it also tones down and clears the skin, eliminating or reducing redness. Yoga, deep breathing, relaxation, and massage are also great solutions. Ideally, you should remove the stressors in your internal and external environment by getting to the root cause of the challenge. Removing stressors is the ultimate long-term solution, and one that contributes most to the balanced life.

## RESILIENCE

If you have seen the movie *Rocky* then you probably recall that you could knock Rocky down, but he would get right back up again. This is resilience at its best. As a youngster, I could easily have given up after being put down multiple times. However, I continually bounced back and recovered.

Some of us are resilient by nature; others are not. Companies, sports teams, and politicians fail and fall, but the ability to recover from fumbles or outright errors and bounce back is a process. Resilience is drawn from strength of character and the will to go on. We have all seen it. Think about a young widow who has young children and whose partner did not return from war. Think about the freak accident that took the lives of an entire family, leaving only the husband/father. Think about the acts of nature that wipe out entire communities. Those with resilience recover more quickly, snap back, and create excitement about the future.

This chapter has addressed the global stress epidemic; the impact of healing environments; the workforce factor; the cost of stress to you, your health, and your employer; and methods of stress reduction. Stress has reached epidemic proportions and the human body's response is constantly challenged. Stress is a part of everyday life: it can promote growth and competency, or it can contribute to adverse effects.

According to New Life Solutions (2013), stress and the related illness, absenteeism, and presenteeism, costs organizations as much as $300 billion annually. Stress contributes to unhealthy behaviors, which contribute to health care costs and lost productivity. Let's face the truth—stress causes you to make many poor lifestyle decisions, and if you can recognize the stressors, address the root cause, and take corrective actions, you can begin the journey toward a life in balance. So, set realistic expectations for yourself. Then, review the solutions offered in this chapter and integrate them within your own life and within your workplace. The time to start is now!

""My grandmother started walking five miles a day when she was sixty. She's ninety-seven now, and we don't know where the heck she is."

—Ellen DeGeneres

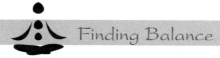 Finding Balance

## AN EXERCISE PLAN

How much time can you commit this week to exercise? Next week? Use the grid to develop a regular schedule. Try to build up to exercise at least 4 to 5 days per week. Vary the type of exercise you do so you do not get bored with your regimen.

|         | M | T | W | Th | F | Sat | Sun |
|---------|---|---|---|----|---|-----|-----|
| Week 1  |   |   |   |    |   |     |     |
| Week 2  |   |   |   |    |   |     |     |
| Week 3  |   |   |   |    |   |     |     |
| Week 4  |   |   |   |    |   |     |     |
| Week 5  |   |   |   |    |   |     |     |
| Week 6  |   |   |   |    |   |     |     |

This might be a good time to schedule that power nap discussed earlier in the chapter.

## TAKE A POWER NAP

To jumpstart the power-nap process, relax all the muscles of your body from the top of your head to your toes. Imagine yourself in a warm and comfortable environment that creates happy, relaxing memories for you, and gently will yourself into a relaxing sleep. Commit to yourself and you will drift into a gentle sleep. You may think drifting into a relaxed state of being at your desk or somewhere else safe and appropriate is impossible, but it will come easily with practice and concentrated effort.

You may question whether you will come out of this phase of sleep in a timely manner, but with practice you will learn to set your own internal alarm clock that will wake you up at the right time. And, when you awaken, you will be refreshed and alive with vigor. Until you become practiced at power napping, set an alarm to remind you to wake up. However, select a gentle alarm bell; being jarred awake will cause you to lose the benefit of the restful feelings from the power nap. Better yet, partner with a friend and watch over each other to be sure you awaken on time.

You may use the power-nap relaxation exercises throughout the day to fully relax your body. Simply relax all of your muscles from head to toe. Try it while sitting at your desk—loosen your neck and shoulders.

## REFLECTIONS

- Maintain a personal environment that sustains you
- Bounce back as needed
- Stay in the present and move forward
- Know when to ask for help and where to get it

# References

American Institute of Stress. (n.d.). Workplace stress. Retrieved from http://www.stress.org/workplace-stress/

American Psychological Society. (2012). Workplace Survey. Retrieved from http://www.apa.org/news/press/releases/phwa/workplace-survey.pdf

Baltra, P., Sharma, A. K., & Khajuria, R. (2013). Probing Lingzhi or Reishi medicinal mushroom Ganoderma lucidum (higher Basidiomycetes): A bitter mushroom with amazing health benefits. *International Journal of Medicinal Mushrooms, 15*(2), 127-143.

Brydon, L., & Steptoe, A. (2005). Stress-induced increase in interleukin-6 and fibrinogen predict ambulatory blood pressure at 3-year follow-up. *Journal of Hypertension, 23*(5), 1001-1007. Retrieved from http://journals.lww.com/jhypertension/Abstract/2005/05000/Stress_induced_increases_in_interleukin_6_and.16.aspx

Chen, T. S., Liou, S. Y., & Chang, Y. L. (2008). Antioxidant evaluation of three adaptogen extracts. *American Journal of Chinese Medicine, 36*(6), 1209-1217.

Fenelon, L., Holcroft, L., & Waters, N. (2009). Contamination of stethoscopes with MRSA and current disinfection practices. *Journal of Hospital Infection, 71*(4), 376-378.

Hansen, C. D., & Andersen, J. H. (2008). Going ill to work–what personal circumstances, attitudes and work-related factors are associated with sickness presenteeism? *Social Science Medicine, 67*(6), 956-964.

Jiang, J., & Sliva, D. (2010). Novel medicinal mushrooms blend suppresses growth and invasiveness of human breast cancer cells. *International Journal of Oncology, 37*(6): 1529-1536.

Kolla, B. P., & Auger, R. R. (2011). Jet lag and shift work sleep disorders: How to help reset the internal clock. *Cleveland Clinic Journal of Medicine, 78*(10), 675-684.

Naska, A., Oikoniomou, E., Trichopoulou, A., Psaltopoulou, T., & Trichopoulos, D. (2007). Siesta in healthy adults and coronary mortality in the general population. *Archives in Internal Medicine, 167*(3), 296-301.

National Institute for Occupational Safety and Health (NIOSH). (n.d.). Stress at work. NIOSH Publication No. 99-101. Retrieved from http://www.cdc.gov/niosh/docs/99-101/

New Life Solutions. (2013). The download on stress. Retrieved from https://www.mequilibrium.com/wp-content/uploads/2013/03/3-1-13-FINAL.pdf

Phillips, A. (2011). A walk in the woods: Evidence builds that time spent in the natural world benefits human health. *American Scientist, 99*(4), 301. Retrieved from http://www.americanscientist.org/issues/pub/a-walk-in-the-woods

Preuss, H. G., Echard, B., Bagchi, D., & Perricone, N. V. (2010). Maitake mushroom extracts ameliorate progressive hypertension and other chronic metabolic perturbations in aging female rats. *International Journal of Medicine Science, 7*(4), 169-180.

Sarnataro, B. R. (n.d.) Top 10 fitness facts: Some things you should know about exercise. WebMD. Retrieved from http://www.webmd.com/fitness-exercise/guide/exercise-benefits

Scott, E. (2008). Sleep benefits: Power napping for increased productivity, stress relief & health. Retrieved from http://stress.about.com/od/lowstresslifestyle/a/powernap.htm

Stephens, S. (2013). Presenteeism—The productivity drain. *HR News Magazine.* Retrieved from http://www.hrnewsmagazine.com/?page_id=681

Steptoe, A., & Marmot, M. G. (2003). The burden of psychosocial adversity and vulnerability in middle-age: Associations of biobehavioral risk factors and quality of life. *Psychosomatic Medicine, 65*(6), 1029-1037.

Stuber, J. (2012). Helping mental health professionals get suicide-prevention training. Retrieved from http://www.rwjf.org/en/blogs/human-capital-blog/2012/04/suicide-prevention-training.html

Towers Watson. (2011/2012). *Staying@Work Stress Survey Report: Pathway to Health and Productivity*. National Business Group on Health.

WebMD. (2014). The effects of stress on your body. Retrieved from http://www.webmd.com/mental-health/effects-of-stress-on-your-body

Widera, E., Chang, A., & Chen, H. L. (2010). Presenteeism: A public health hazard. *Journal of General Internal Medicine, 25*(11), 1244-1247. Retrieved from http://www.ncbi.nlm.nih.gov/pmc/articles/PMC2947637/

*"The biggest adventure you can ever take is to live the life of your dreams."*

—Oprah Winfrey

# 4

# FOCUS AND BEGIN TO DREAM AGAIN

*—Sharon M. Weinstein, MS, RN, CRNI, FACW, FAAN*

A chaotic life can easily distract you from your focus. How many times in a day do you find yourself in a room, knowing you were there for a reason, but unable to remember the reason you went there? Or at the end of the day, with a heavy sigh, do you look over your to-do list from that morning and realize you barely made a dent in your list? We joke and attribute these problems to old age, but even the young do this. More likely it is a difficulty in maintaining focus.

## FOCUS

We live in an age of distraction, and, simply put, *focus* is about finding simplicity within this age. If you are familiar with the concept of emotional intelligence, you may also be aware of author Daniel Goleman's (2013) concept of focus as today's scarcest resource and the secret to high performance as well as fulfillment. Navarro (2010) suggests that you ask yourself, "What would I need to focus on to feel this way?" The question forces you to stop thinking about the things that are draining you and to acknowledge that there are things you can focus on that will provide more mental and emotional energy.

## What Focus Is and Why It's Important

Focus is the thing that keeps us on track. It's what we need when we have a goal to achieve. We keep *focused* on doing what we need to do to accomplish the tasks that cumulatively make up the goal. Focus is also an ability to remain undistracted. It is what we use to intently pursue a goal, such as running the Boston Marathon, studying for exams, writing a paper, or creating artwork. It is this kind of focus that is the source of the "aha" moment we hope for when seeking solutions and setting goals.

Have you ever experienced an aha moment, or a sudden insight (Kounios & Beeman, 2009)? We all have, and sometimes I have wondered why it took me so long to "get it." The aha moment is a moment of clarity when you gain wisdom that may change your life. Big or small, funny or sad, these moments are unique, personal, and sometimes well worth sharing. Merriam-Webster included the word *aha* in the dictionary as a result of Oprah Winfrey's reference to the word. (*US Weekly* Staff, 2012). Oprah says, "I always love those moments when I sit down to talk to somebody and they say something that makes me look at life or a situation in a completely different way. And I say, 'Aha! I get it!' Light bulb… and the little hairs on your arm stand up. That is an aha moment."

Getting to that aha moment of achievement or recognition includes the knowledge of how to define *your* path and work *your* plan. In 2012, *Forbes* magazine published an informal study on aha moments, and this is my favorite: "No one—not your mother, your clients or the vendors you're working with—wants to tell you 'No' when you ask for something; most people want to find a way to tell you 'Yes'" (Hall, 2012). My aha moment was when I realized this and started asking for what I wanted in life. I truly believe in asking for what you want in life. That became reality when I proposed to my husband on our fifth date, and we were married on the tenth day after we had met. What closed the deal for me? It was the very first phone call, which lasted 3 hours, in which he described his amazing family. Although he was an only child, and his dad had passed when he (my husband) was just 14, he depicted a family of which I wanted to be a part. And, so, I asked by simply focusing and stating, "I'm not working on Wednesday. Would you like to get married?" The rest is history!

"The first time someone shows you who they are, believe them."

—Maya Angelou

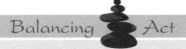

Balancing Act

## THE SPELLING BEE

Our son, at age 12, was preparing for the National Spelling Bee. He was always a good speller, but he focused on the fact that in order to win the prize, which was a computer, he would need to out-spell all other contestants. Working with his coach, an English teacher, he accumulated all of the books used in previous years and a list of "difficult" words Our son strategized on how many words he would have to study per night, over a one-year period, in order to win the prize. I worked with him on a nightly basis, and our goal was to cover 200 words per night. He's blessed with a photographic memory, and consequently he gave me many aha moments. For example, I would say "antimacassar" and he would say, "Is that page 3, the third column, fourth word?" Of course, he was correct—he was focused. He not only remembered the words as they appeared on the written page, but he was able to tell me the origin, meaning, and spell each word accurately.

The qualifying rounds for Nationals were conducted at Trinity University, where he was seated behind a young boy from a small town in Texas. The boy said, "When I am finished here, my dad is going to take me fishing." Our son replied, "When I am finished here, I am going to go home and play with my new computer." Both boys were committed to a goal; both were focused, but our son was also focused on the prize. He went on to win the San Antonio Spelling Bee—and the computer.

When we arrived in Washington, D.C., we were staggered by the numbers of winners from cities and states across the country, all of whom were good spellers. Although all of the participants were focused on the Spelling Bee itself, many switched gears and focused on the excitement of their first airplane flight and the chance to see history come alive through the monuments and treasures of the nation's capital. Many of these contestants who didn't make it through the first and second rounds went on sightseeing trips and took advantage of the opportunity for continuous learning through the sights and sounds of Washington, D.C. Our son maintained his focus with a strong sense of balance, designating certain hours of the day for review of the words and other time slots for sightseeing. This, for me, was an aha moment: A lesson from a 12-year-old boy on how to maintain balance in one's life.

## THE ROCK WALL

And, now, fast forward to my son's son—the boy who made me a grandmother! Let's call him "A." When my son's family was on a Disney cruise, our grandson wanted his dad to climb the rock wall. Our son looked at the wall, which was fairly high, and then at the water surrounding the cruise ship. He thought to himself, "There is no way that I am going to climb that wall." But A, who was 3 at the time, was insistent. So, our son did what any good dad would do. He slipped a Spiderman action figure into his pocket, and he climbed the wall. When he descended, A clapped his hands with joy and said, "Daddy, you did it; you did it." Our son, always Mr. Integrity, wanted to share the story of how he did it, and as he was about to do so, A said, "Daddy, I know how you did it—you believed in yourself." Why is it that a 3 year old gets it, whereas sometimes we adults do not?

## WHEN LIFE COMES INTO FOCUS

You cannot predict when you will have an aha moment. Sometimes it takes days and hours of focus, and sometimes only a few minutes. Sometimes you have to focus on something for much longer, and the aha moment evolves through trial and error and contributions from external sources.

Focus is facilitated through good health. Health is about mind and body. If your consciousness is disturbed, then your body will be, too. If you feel uptight, your body will be tense and it will be difficult to focus.

How can you keep your focus so that you experience more aha moments? Consider the following strategies:

- Be centered.
- Tap into your creative side.
- Keep the "main thing" the main thing.
- Set goals and write them down.
- Find your passion.

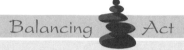

Balancing Act

## AN AHA MOMENT: ARCHIMEDES IN THE BATH

The story of Archimedes in the bath illustrates a perfect aha moment. The king, Hiero, requested a special crown be made and delivered a certain weight in gold to the crown maker. Upon receiving his crown, Hiero had doubts about whether the crown maker had replaced some of the gold with an equal weight of another metal and kept the extra gold for himself. The king asked Archimedes to prove the content of the crown.

As Archimedes submerged himself in his bath, he was suddenly struck with the observation that his body weight displaced the water in the tub. Taking this as the beginning of his discovery, it is said that he made two masses of the same weight as the crown, one of gold and the other of silver. After making them, he filled a large vessel to the brim with water and dropped the mass of silver into it. As much water ran out as was equal in bulk to that of the silver sunk in the vessel. Then he removed the silver mass from the vessel and poured back the lost quantity of water, using a pint measure, until it was level with the brim as it had been before. Thus he found the weight of silver corresponding to a definite quantity of water.

Archimedes then dropped the mass of gold into the full vessel and again measured the amount of water that was displaced. He found that less water was lost with the gold mass than had been lost with the silver mass. In other words, a mass of gold lacks bulk compared to a mass of silver of the same weight.

Finally, filling the vessel again and dropping the crown into the same quantity of water, Archimedes found that more water ran over for the crown than for the mass of gold of the same weight. Based on the fact that more water was lost when the crown was submerged than when the mass of gold was submerged, he reasoned that the crown maker has mixed silver with the gold, which made the theft of the contractor perfectly clear.

# BE CENTERED

Being centered means not letting yourself be overshadowed by what's going on around you. If you're not centered, you will be like a leaf in the wind, at the mercy of circumstance; you will be out of focus. Think about the concept of avoiding distractions, those things that get in the way. You may even relate it to a voice in your head that is telling you one thing when you know that you need to concentrate and finish the task at hand. That little voice can destroy your ability to be centered. More than willpower, and certainly much more than motivation, being centered is the ability to cling to your goals.

What can you do to remain centered? You can visualize the outcome you desire; you can feel the result subconsciously; your can have faith that it will turn out as expected; and you can keep your eyes and heart focused on how you add value to the world each day. You can keep your eye on the ball!

*"I was brought up to believe that the only thing worth doing was to add to the sum of accurate information in this world."*

—Margaret Mead

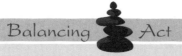

Balancing Act

## KEEPING YOUR EYE ON THE BALL

Our grandson, A, had been learning how to hit a ball, and he wanted
to be really good at it. One lesson my son and husband taught was,
"A, keep your eye on the ball." One day, we looked at A, and he
had a softball up against his eye. We asked what he was doing, and
he replied, "I am keeping my eye on the ball." He was centered; he
made a decision. Learning how to make successful decisions in life
is a critical lesson. You've got to do it, rather than just read or think
about it. Work/life balance requires us to keep the edge. Whether in
softball or a business interest, keep your eye on the ball and your life
in balance.

During aha moments, you are charged up and your mind is working
optimally. During those moments, you can be all that you wish to be—
creative, centered, focused. One of the most important ladders leading to
the top is knowledge. The more you know, the more prepared your mind,
and the higher you can move. You need to make sure that your mind is
prepared and that you are focused. When you are centered, you are more
receptive to new ideas and knowledge.

# TAP INTO YOUR CREATIVE SIDE

Imagination is seeing things not as they are, but as they could be. I have
had the privilege of living in many cities, states, and, for a short time, other
countries. The concept of house hunting is not new to me. Over the years,
before online searches of potential properties in the right school districts
with the right soccer teams, I visited thousands of homes. Fortunately, I
was able to imagine what the homes would look like with my own special
touches of paint, wall covering, carpeting, and furnishings. I could easily
identify those homes that had potential. When we settled on a property,
I used a four-step process to tap into my creative soul—quite deeply at

times—to bring these houses to life and make them our homes. The four steps are

1. Preparation
2. Incubation
3. Illumination
4. Implementation.

Those four steps may easily be transferred into many daily activities. When you approach a new project, you need to *prepare* by gathering information and resources. You then *incubate* the idea, letting your subconscious mind play with the information. Next, you experience the aha moment, *illuminating* the idea and bringing it to life. And finally, you *implement*, either by doing or not doing a certain action or strategy. John Maxwell once said, "Lots of folks have great ideas in the shower, but they seem to lose them when they dry off." Is that you?

"Over the years I have developed a picture of what a human being living humanely is like. She is a person who understands, values, and develops her body, finding it beautiful and useful; a person who is real and is willing to take risks, to be creative, to manifest competence, to change when the situation calls for it, and to find ways to accommodate to what is new and different, keeping that part of the old that is still useful and discarding what is not.""

–Virginia Satir

Try thinking about all the times in your career when you went through these steps to help a patient. One example is a nurse who wanted to help a lonely male resident at a long-term care facility. She prepared by gathering information about the man, his family (who were all living out of state), his past hobbies (writing, but he could no longer use a keyboard or pen), and past experiences (teaching). She let her information incubate until she had an aha moment: The man narrated stories about his family into a tape recorder, sent them to his family, who made their own tapes and sent them back. He also started teaching other residents how to write their own memoirs.

## Balancing Act

### FIND YOUR MOTIVATION

All kinds of studies have been made regarding motivation. Self-determination theory is based on human motivation, development, and wellness, according to Deci and Ryan (2008). What is it that motivates people to do the things they do, live the way they live, achieve the goals they achieve? The root of the word motivation is *move*, and movement is change. Ask yourself the following questions: Are you moving forward or standing still? Do you love your work? Do you love your career? Do you have good personal relationships? Is your attitude in check? Are you in balance?

We often lock the doors to our comfort zones so that we can't get to growth, discovery, and adventure. Unlock those doors and focus on the prize. We don't remember days as much as we remember moments. Make the aha moments count!

# KEEP THE "MAIN THING" THE MAIN THING

What does that mean to you? An aha moment is something you can't plan; it just happens. It is a joy to be there when that moment occurs for someone you know.

In nursing, we have many aha moments. For example, when you discovered that the first bed bath is not that difficult. As a new graduate, when you discovered the passion of your role within the profession. As a nurse educator, when you saw the smile on the face of a student and realized that he or she had connected the dots and that the complex process that you just explained was quite simple after all. As a nursing administrator, when you realized that you had met your expectations for the organization and fulfilled your professional and personal goals.

The aha moment often drives us to the main thing; it is a moment of sudden realization that we are on track, or that we need to switch gears to reach our goals. Consider the aha moment a paradigm shift or a computer reboot. Perhaps it offers sudden insight or a perspective you had not previously considered. You are seeking new ways of doing things, rather than the same old way that has always worked. Yet, you still need to remain focused on the target. No matter who you are or where you work, you need to keep the main thing the main thing. The type of work does not matter, nor does the setting in which you work. Whether you are a nurse, a teacher, a production worker, an IT expert, a publisher, or a public figure—the main thing remains the main thing. Don't stray from the goal; identify creative ways to reach the target faster and better. Some how-to's on keeping the main thing the main thing include:

- Evaluate where you are at present (how do you spend your time and with whom).
- Make the "main thing" a daily target, part of your daily life by focusing on the goal (add the goal to your calendar).
- Create a list of things that might create barriers (if something deters you, perhaps you should eliminate that barrier).
- If you are working as a team, get input from all team members (it is probably larger than anything that one can accomplish alone).

"When one door of happiness closes, another opens, but often we took so long at the closed door that we do not see the one that has been opened up for us."

—Helen Keller

# GOAL SETTING WITH FOCUS IN MIND

At the start of every year, people all across the world set goals or resolutions for the New Year. Many of these resolutions are promises that all-too-often get broken—to lose 10 pounds, to increase exercise, to give up one bad habit or another, and to live a better life. Many of these resolutions are actually goals that require commitments and action plans for success.

Yes, there are those of us who set goals, state affirmations, get motivated, and do not succeed. Are you one of them? In reality, a very small percentage of people actually set purposeful goals and follow them through.

It has often been said that the line that separates winning from losing is as fine as a razor's edge. One may *see* an opportunity and the other may *seize* an opportunity. You learned the distinction between winning and losing from a very young age. You learned the difference between being chosen for teams and being left out or forgotten. So how do you separate the winners from the losers now? Are you not all winners simply by competing? How do some see an opportunity and consider it, while others see it and eagerly grasp that chance, that gold ring, that opportunity of a lifetime?

Setting goals gives your life direction, not unlike those New Year's resolutions. Goal setting is a powerful process for realizing your dreams; by setting precise goals, you can measure your progress, reward yourself for small steps along the way, and celebrate your successes.

Opportunity presents itself—perhaps it is a business offer, a writing or speaking assignment, or a relocation. Will you see or seize? *Seize* is an action verb; it requires you to take action…and action will result in a growth experience, financial rewards, or continuous learning. Think about the process of "trying" as opposed to "doing." Years ago, there were two major car rental companies in America. One of them tried (Avis), while the other did (Hertz). Then, along came Enterprise, and while Avis and Hertz were trying to outdo one another with advertisements, Enterprise saw an opportunity, seized it, and became the most prolific car rental company we have ever seen.

*"Sometimes opportunities float right past your nose. Work hard, apply yourself, and be ready. When an opportunity comes you can grab it."*

—Julie Andrews Edwards

# FIND YOUR PASSION—VISUALLY

Your passion is what separates ordinary from extraordinary. Take the time to discover your passions by creating a list of what you like to do, those you admire most, and where you would like to travel. If you can see it, you can believe it—and the same is true of your passions. If you can visualize them, you are more likely to reach them.

Chapter 12 discusses the use of a vision board as a planning tool in great detail. The board helps you to define your purpose, add clarity to your desires, and add feeling to your vision. It helps to identify your succession plan—from a job, a professional society, or a position within a networking group. The key in succession management is to create a match between the company or group's future needs and the aspirations of individual employees or members. In order to reach your goal, you need a plan, and a vision board starts the process; it is a blueprint for success.

# A BLUEPRINT FOR SUCCESS

Human beings come into this world to do particular work. Those of us in the health professions are here to do special work. Teachers provide a special gift to mold young minds. The work is our purpose, and each is specific to the person. Focus is a blueprint for success, and by being focused on the goal, you position yourself for success.

Search is an integral part of the process. Finding out who you are is one of the key steps in finding out what you are here to do. It might be the most important step in keeping you focused. Who are you as a nursing professional? Where is your blueprint for success?

# THE DREAM

*"It does not do to dwell on dreams and forget to live."*
—J. K. Rowling

Today, somewhere, someone is going to go back to school to improve his or her life. Someone is going to look in the mirror and see a need to lose a little weight, which will spur the decision to become healthy. Someone will run a first marathon. Someone, somewhere, is going to set out on a pathway to success and reach beyond dreams to change lives.

## EXAMPLES OF DREAMERS WHO HAVE CREATED CHANGE IN THE WORLD

Often, people dream big dreams and have great aspirations. These are waking dreams, planned-for dreams—the kind of dreams sometimes referred to as ambition. You might know the names of many successful dreamers—those whose actions made their dreams come true—because you see them frequently in the media. Here are some examples:

- Barack Obama is the first African-American elected to be president of the United States.
- The Chicago Blackhawks hockey team led the season in 2013 and went on to win the prized Stanley Cup by scoring two goals within 17 seconds during the last minute and 37 seconds of the game.
- Meryl Davis and Charlie White, 2014 ice dancing gold medalists at the Sochi Olympics, gave the United States its first ice

dancing medal. Meryl was diagnosed with dyslexia in the third grade and struggled with reading until the eleventh grade. Her learning disability did not hold her back from pursuing her life's purpose—skating.

- Michael Phelps has won 18 gold Olympic medals, the most by any Olympian in history.

- Shannon Miller is the only American to rank among the Top 10 All-Time gymnasts. She's also the only female athlete to be inducted into the U.S. Olympic Hall of Fame (twice, no less)!

- Oprah Winfrey is an internationally syndicated talk-show host and media mogul who is ranked among the most powerful people in history.

- Yao Ming is the first Chinese National Basketball Association (NBA) star.

- Bill Gates is the founder of Microsoft and a billionaire philanthropist.

- Steve Jobs was the founder of Apple. His definition of focus was the ability to say "no."

This list could go on and on. We all have heroes or heroines who inspire and motivate us and not all of them make the evening news or even their local weekly newspapers. These people are no less successful as dreamers because they haven't become the president of the United States or won 18 Olympic gold medals. What makes someone a dreamer is the ability to envision a possibility for the future and then to make that vision a reality, one step at a time.

## BEGIN TO DREAM YOUR DREAM

*"He who robs us of our dreams robs us of our life."*
—Virgina Woolf

I am a dreamer. With calm confidence, I encourage others, through my own story, to thrive and survive! Forget tragedy and setbacks. Forget the fact that you were told you would never amount to anything! I can inspire you to live an exquisite life, believe in yourself, embrace vulnerability, and live your dreams!

We're able to live our dreams by knowing our *why*. Why start with *why*? The goal is not to fix the things that aren't working. Instead, focus on and amplify the things that do work in your life.   You can live your life, dream your dreams, share your successes, and achieve more if you remind yourself to know your why, believe in your dreams, visualize those dreams, expect a hard way ahead, and take one bite at a time. There is no such thing as an impossible dream. Someone, somewhere, is going to set out on a pathway to success and reach beyond dreams to change lives. Let that someone be you!

## THE TIPPING POINT

Malcolm Gladwell, in his compelling book *The Tipping Point*, (2002) says that change is possible; people or social institutions can radically transform their behavior in the face of the right impetus. This is the ultimate "tipping point," and the author provides compelling examples of a number of forces coming together—many of which appeared small or inconsequential—that result in a large-scale change. For example, there was a tipping point for violent crime in New York in the 1990s, as well as a tipping point for the reemergence of Hush Puppies, much like the tipping point for the introduction of new technologies.

Within our careers as nurses, we have many examples of *tipping points*. Advocacy, interprofessional collaboration and mentorship, transforming healthcare, and best practices are all tipping points. Each of these movements could have failed had they not had their own *salesmen* and *connectors*, the terms Gladwell uses to describe those with vast networks of people in various personal and professionals pools who hear new ideas, talk about them, and share them. Think of the connectors in your practice, in your work, in your profession. Think about what sets them apart from others. What makes them connectors who facilitate the success of others as they change lives?

## Nursing's Dreamers

The nursing profession has dreamers of its own. The list may begin with Florence Nightingale and extend to include others who have changed the face of our profession. I consider many of my nurse colleagues from the new independent states of the former Soviet Union and Central and Eastern European countries to be dreamers. They had a vision; they followed their passions; and they realized their dreams. In the process, they set the standard for others to follow.

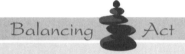

Balancing Act

## Who Are Your Dreamers?

Martin Luther King's famous "I Have a Dream" speech has been changing people's lives across America and the world ever since he uttered those four powerful words. And although his life came to an early tragic end, his family and his followers have kept his dream alive.

Within the healthcare arena, we are often called upon to build coalitions; it is an integral part of the survival process. Wendy Kopp, founder and president of Teach for America, is a coalition builder and someone from whom we can learn. "She proposed the idea for Teach For America in her Princeton University undergraduate thesis in 1989. In 1990, a charter corps of 500 committed recent college graduates joined Teach For America and began fueling the movement to eliminate educational inequity. Since then, nearly 33,000 participants have reached more than 3 million children nationwide during their two-year teaching commitments. They have sustained their commitment as alumni, working within education and across all sectors to help ensure that children growing up in low-income communities get an excellent education" (Teach For America, 2014, para. 1). Her highly developed leadership skills and use of social strategies led to the creation of a privately funded, nonprofit organization with 15 offices. Kopp transformed the public education system at three levels: state policy, district teaching, and national public awareness. Kopp, formerly a "doer" herself, has grown tremendously, empowering others along the way. She, like Dr. King, had a dream. She made this dream a reality. In the process, Teach for America, Inc. has become a holding company for three other programs—Teach, Learning Project, and Teach for America—that are changing the lives of people across the United States.

Think about some dreamers—those who have risen through the ranks and achieved great things. Write their names and their success stories.

Next, create your own dream inventory. Dreams may be good or bad. Many people share universal dreams. Some examples include:

- Falling in front of a car or train
- Suffering natural disasters
- Flying in a plane
- Appearing naked in public
- Losing your teeth
- Finding or losing money

You may have experienced some of these dreams as a child, and you may have wondered what they meant. This list includes a number of threatening dreams—you may consider them nightmares. A good way to deal with them is to reverse them—make them positive things that happen to you, such as:

- Saving someone from in front of a car or train
- Surviving a natural disaster and savings others
- Piloting a plane to a safe landing

You get the idea! You can actually rescript, reenact, and rehearse the dreams to become something favorable and memorable. You can use storyboards, visuals, or art to retell your dreams.

## DEFINING YOUR DREAMS

You may have a lot of aspirations that you consider dreams. Maybe you dream about a new car, a better job, a nice house, a long-term relationship, time and money to travel the world, time and money to help others, a new career, or winning the lottery. Are all of these dreams? Goals, maybe, but it's doubtful they are all dreams. How do you tell the difference? The following is a quick brainstorming exercise you can do to cull the goals (or wants) from the dreams. Ask yourself the following questions and write down the answer as quickly as possible. Don't think about them too much.

What would you do if…

- You won $1 million?
- You had to return to college to get a four-year degree?
- You lost your present job?
- You had a disability that prevented you from walking?
- You won $1,000 a week for life?
- You had 6 months to live?

These questions should force you to look behind what you might assume to be your dream. For example, you might assume that your dream is to have lots of money—but what do you want from that money? What do you want to do with your time? With whom do you want to spend your time?

*"What you can do, or dream you can, begin it. Boldness has genius, power, and magic in it."*

—Goethe

## MOVING FORWARD TOWARD YOUR DREAMS

Have you ever had inventor's remorse in the hardware or home store upon seeing some clever invention—or remake of an old invention—that you had perhaps contemplated years before? Although you might have had the idea, someone else had the idea as well, but saw it through to fruition; for him or her it became a "dream come true." The inventor followed his or her passion and created something, whereas you merely thought about it and then let it go. The other person made the idea become a reality, just as Thomas Edison and the Wright brothers did.

That's not to say putting your dreams into action is always easy. There are many hurdles and roadblocks you have to surmount. When I worked in the former Soviet Union on healthcare projects with many of my nurse colleagues from across North America, we learned some hard lessons. When a contract needed to be signed or work needed to be done on a hospital renovation project, we were repeatedly reminded that although anything is possible, not everything is probable. The *dream* was to rebuild the hospital to international standards of quality. It was imperative to keep the dream foremost in our thoughts while we struggled with all the details that had to come together to make that dream come true. We realized our dreams through persistence and tenacity. So, be persistent and reap the benefits. By building your dream—helping your dream to come to life, no matter what it may be—you build yourself.

Do the following things to move toward your goals:

- Believe in your dream. Make sure it's something you want to, and can, pour your heart into.

- Visualize your dream. Visualizing your dream energizes you because you can see how the world changes for the better and how people (including you) live a happier life because of your dream.

- Expect a hard way ahead. Enough said.

- Take one bite at a time. Set reasonable and achievable goals. It's no good to create hurdles so high you will inevitably fail. Set the first goals low enough that you are sure to achieve them, and set each successive series of goals more aggressively as you gain confidence in moving toward the goal.

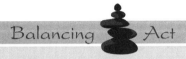

Balancing Act

# DREAMING OF A FUTURE THAT COULD BE

As a young girl growing up in an abusive household, I often dreamed of what could be. I looked at the relationships my friends had with their parents and families and wished I could have that in my life. I knew that I could be better, that I could do better, and at age 14 I set out on a mission to prove it.

*"Every great dream begins with a dreamer. Always remember, you have within you the strength, the patience, and the passion to reach for the stars to change the world. "*

—Harriet Tubman

My healthcare career began then. I started volunteering at age 14, first in a hospital morgue and then on the patient care units. At the same time, I found as many jobs as possible to generate income. The jobs were varied—from assisting an accountant with the daily receipts of a number of local food establishments to babysitting and more. I worked long hours, and I worked hard. I developed a strong work ethic from my affiliation with the accountant. He taught me the importance of completing a task in order to realize my goals. He served as a referral for me when I applied to nursing school, and he became a lifelong friend and mentor.

I knew I needed a good education to realize my dreams, and I saw nursing as the vehicle to help me achieve them. Although my initial program was only 3 years, leading to a diploma, I graduated with honors and went on to complete bachelor's and master's degrees on a continuum of learning that has not yet stopped.

I was fortunate to have had a role model who believed in me and my ability and who helped me to understand the value of dreams.

## SUPPORTING YOUR DREAMS?

Each and every day, people across the country and around the world are living their dreams. Are you one of them? You may think that your dreams are out of reach and that it is impossible. But, people prove every day that someone is going to get healthy, strong, smart, rich, famous, and hopefully along the way improve their lives.

*"So many of our dreams at first seem impossible; then they seem improbable, and then, when we summon the will, they soon become inevitable."*

*—Christopher Reeve*

Don't allow self-doubt to interfere with your success. There is no such thing as an impossible dream. There are only dreams without action steps that will make them realities. Make sure you support your dream. Share the dream and your plan with loved ones. Make sure you have people who can offer moral support on low days.

*"You may say I'm a dreamer, but I'm not the only one."*

*—John Lennon*

We began this chapter with focus—what it is and why we need it. We transitioned into being centered, the necessity to keep the main thing the main thing, and goal setting. Throughout this chapter, we have discussed the concept of dreams. Examples defined dreamers—those who have realized their dreams and those who are in the process. You were asked to identify your own dreams and to move forward toward them.

Focus is the entry point; it is a beginning. It provides the opportunity to focus on what is most important, and then to give your dreams a chance!

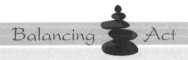

## GIVE DREAMS A CHANCE

Many people experience their best dreams during the day, but the nights can yield ideas and inspiration, too.

Dreams generally are associated with the sleep cycle, and it is during rapid eye movement (REM 5) sleep that we dream most deeply. One sleep cycle comprises five stages in the sleep cycle, including delta, or the first 5 to 10 minutes when you are falling asleep. The sleep cycle repeats itself about an average of four to five times per night, but it may repeat as many as seven times. Thus, you can see how a person has several different dreams in one night. Most people, however, only remember dreams that occur closer toward the morning when they are about to wake up. Just because you can't remember other dreams does not mean that they never happened. Some people swear on the fact that they simply do not dream; in reality, they just don't remember their dreams. The actual sleep cycle is addressed as stages of sleep (Institute of Medicine, 2006). See Chapter 9 for more information.

*Stage 1*: This is known as Delta One, and everyone has experienced it. For example, when your eyes begin to droop while you're driving or sitting in a classroom. This is the beginning of the sleep cycle.

*Stage 2*. You are entering into light sleep. This stage is characterized by nonrapid eye movements (NREM), muscle relaxation, lowered body temperature, and slowed heart rate. The body is preparing to enter into deep sleep.

*Stage 3:* Also characterized by NREM, this stage is characterized by a further drop in body temperature and relaxation of the muscles. The body's immune system goes to work on repairing the day's damage, the endocrine glands secrete growth hormone, and blood is sent to the muscles to be reconditioned. In this stage, you are completely asleep.

*Stage 4*: Still in the NREM stage, this is a still deeper sleep. Your metabolic levels are extremely slow.

*Stage 5*: In this stage of sleep, your eyes move back and forth erratically. Referred to as REM sleep or delta sleep, this stage occurs at about 90 to 100 minutes after the onset of sleep. Your blood pressure rises, heart rate speeds up, respiration becomes erratic, and brain activity increases. Your involuntary muscles also become paralyzed. This stage is the most restorative part of sleep. Your mind is being revitalized and emotions are being fine-tuned. The majority of your dreaming occurs in this stage.

Do you dream? Do you even sleep? A number of nurse researchers have spent their careers studying the sleep patterns of men and women. Mid-afternoon tiredness may be alleviated with a glass of water; hydration is critical. Tips to fight insomnia include:

- Avoid alcohol, caffeine, and heavy, spicy, or sugary foods 4 to 6 hours before sleep

- Stick to a daily routine

- Exercise regularly

- Block out distractions

- Practice relaxation techniques

- Drink a cup of Lingzhi tea before bed

- Establish presleep rituals

- Stay hydrated, especially during afternoon periods of tiredness

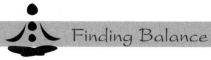 Finding Balance

## REFLECTIONS

- What were your daydreams as a child?

- What are three dreams that you have accomplished in your life? Write them down. What efforts contributed to the accomplishment of those dreams?

- What are you dreaming about doing right now that you aren't accomplishing?

- What are the barriers to achieving your current dream? Make a list and then develop a plan for working through each one.

# References

Deci, E. L., & Ryan, R. M. (2008). Self-determination theory: A macrotheory of human motivation, development, and health. *Canadian Psychology, 49*(3): 182-185.

Gladwell, M. (2002). *The tipping point: How little things can make a big difference.* Boston, MA: Little, Brown & Co.

Goleman, D. (2013). *Focus: The hidden driver of excellence.* New York: HarperCollins.

Hall, A. (2012, October 15). 100 founders share their top 'aha' moments—guess how many jobs they've created so far? [Web log post] Retrieved from www.forbes.com/sites/alanhall/2012/10/15/100-founders-share-their-top-aha-moments-guess-how-many-jobs-theyve-created-so-far/

Institute of Medicine Committee on Sleep Medicine and Research. (2006). Sleep physiology. In H. R. Colten and B. M. Altevogt (Eds.), *Sleep Disorders and Sleep Deprivation: An Unmet Public Health Problem.* Washington, DC: National Academies Press. Retrieved from http://www.ncbi.nlm.nih.gov/books/NBK19956/

Kounios, J., & Beeman, M. (2009). The aha! moment: the cognitive neuroscience of insight. *Current Directions in Psychological Science, 18*(4): 210–216

Navarro, D. (2010). How to stay focused. [Web log post] Retrieved from http://www.rockyourday.com/how-to-stay-focused

Teach For America. (2014). Our history. Retrieved from http://www.teachforamerica.org/our-organization/our-history

*US Weekly* Staff. (2012). Oprah's "Aha Moment" added to Merriam-Webster dictionary. *US Weekly.* Retrieved from http://www.usmagazine.com/celebrity-news/news/oprahs-aha-moment-added-to-merriam-webster-dictionary-2012168

*"The past, the present and the future are really one: they are today."*

—Harriet Beecher Stowe

# 5

# GET ENGAGED… IN YOUR LIFE

*—Marla Vannucci, PhD*

Everyone has had the experience of spacing out while driving. We get lost in our thoughts and all of a sudden have reached our destination, or we wind up at the office on a non-work day because we are so used to driving that route. Our bodies are constructed to perform many functions on autopilot, and well-learned tasks in particular do not require our full mental participation. Especially when experiences or activities are expected or routinized, we may feel as if we can complete these tasks "in our sleep." Ironically, we can become so good at certain tasks, in our lives and at work, that we do not need to pay attention in order to complete these tasks effectively. Yet, inattention can lead to errors or mistakes with consequences that range from small to devastating. Whereas novel activities capture our attention easily because we must concentrate to perform well, we may need to exert extra effort to focus on routine or regular tasks in which errors have significant negative results. Even more importantly, in living our lives on autopilot, we may rob ourselves of moments of creativity, joy, purpose, and balance that would be experienced through greater engagement.

# WHAT IS ENGAGEMENT?

I am a clinical psychologist, and when my patients discuss their experiences of depression, they often describe feeling as if they are in a fog or living in a cloud. One particularly distressed patient explained, "I feel like I can't touch my life." Disconnectedness, although a hallmark of some forms of depression, is not unique to depression. In the busy modern age of instant accessibility, for many of us life can feel like a to-do list rather than an experience.

The positive psychology movement, formed officially in the late 1990s, focuses on understanding happiness, resilience, well-being, and optimism (Seligman & Peterson, 2003). Positive psychology suggests that happiness comes not from indulging personal wants and not simply from positive thinking, but rather from two key elements: 1) engagement in daily life, and 2) finding meaning and purpose (Duckworth, Steen, & Seligman, 2005). You can find a discussion of purpose and meaning in Chapter 1. This chapter discusses engagement and how it can help you to achieve greater balance, well-being, productivity, and satisfaction in your life.

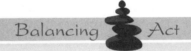

Balancing Act

## AN EXAMPLE OF ENGAGED HAPPINESS

Before I had my son, I struggled to be in the moment. After he was born, I quickly realized that when I was caring for him, I could only focus on him in order to care for his needs adequately. Splitting my attention meant I did nothing well. At first this was a great challenge for me because I was constantly thinking about what else needed to be done. I have worked to be fully present in moments of closeness with him, such as our "morning snuggle." Rather than watching the clock to see if I'm going to be late, hurrying him to get dressed, or thinking about the dishes in the sink, I simply sit in the moment of holding him. Part of this effort came from realizing that his needs are immediate and cannot be added to the to-do list, but also from the knowledge that he would not always want to snuggle with me, so I needed to enjoy it while it lasted. Forcing myself to focus on what I was doing with him in the moment rather than what should happen next was difficult; yet in working to be present with him, I now feel joy, contentment, and peace that set a much more pleasant tone for us to start our day than my trying to do a million things at once. When I'm feeling stressed out during the day, I think back on the morning snuggle and how nice it felt, and it grounds me.

## ASSESSING YOUR ENGAGEMENT

- Think about moments in your life when you feel happiness or satisfaction with yourself and your life. What are you doing when you experience contentment? Are you working, participating in a hobby, by yourself, or with others?

- How engaged are you in your life right now? In what activities at work and in your life do you typically find yourself on autopilot, completing the task almost without noticing? How does a lack of engagement affect your performance in these activities?

- Are there moments at work and in your life in which you are fully present, conscious, and in the moment? These are moments in which you may find that you are able to think quickly on your feet.

- Lastly, is there an activity at work or in your life in which you become completely immersed, where you do not notice time passing, but you feel challenged and engaged?

If you imagine that engagement is a coin, experiences of acute, in-the-moment self-awareness and losing oneself in deep immersion are the two sides of that coin.

# FLEXIBILITY AND THE DEFAULT POSITION

Martin Seligman, who is often credited with the establishment of positive psychology, was initially well known for his learned helplessness theory of depression. Early on, Seligman suggested that depression can stem from feeling that our efforts in life are futile and that we are unable to make change in our lives (Seligman, 1975). The concept of engagement flows naturally from Seligman's earlier ideas. Being more present enables us to make changes and to have power and influence in our own lives. In psychotherapy, self-awareness is often the first step required to make a life change. Without self-awareness, how can we know what to change?

With anything new we attempt to integrate into our lives, it can be easy to focus on the new habit or behavior for a short period of time and then abandon it. Although some people practice engagement in a formal way, you can also practice it in your everyday life, without adding anything to your to-do list. Engagement involves a new way of thinking and perceiving yourself and, eventually, a new way of being in your world. A patient of mine once referred to changing habits as "setting a new default." Her default position was not to exercise each day, so riding her bike to work required an active change out of her default position. She decided that riding her bike each day would become her new default. Engagement behavior can become a new default position over time; however, to begin, we focus on practicing engagement in small moments rather than approaching engagement as a radical behavior change.

As a psychotherapist and teacher of future psychologists, I am able to feel that I am helping others every day. However, helping is not synonymous with engagement. When I am not fully engaged in my therapy office or in my classroom, and when I run on autopilot, I feel less satisfaction and contentment. I am more likely to make mistakes and to experience burnout. When I am fully present with my clients, I feel alive, productive, and even joyful. The activities in my workday may be the same from one day to the next, but my level of engagement determines my experience during my day, my feelings about my day, and my energy level at the end of the day.

You might feel hesitant about putting time and energy into yourself and your own well-being. Similarly, my patients on occasion express ambivalence about being in therapy, believing that focusing on them seems self-centered or indulgent. Self-awareness is quite different from self-consciousness, which is what we experience when we are critiquing ourselves throughout the day or ruminating about events that have already happened. Self-consciousness makes our lives smaller, limiting our choices and our flexibility in the world. Self-awareness, on the other hand, makes our lives bigger and opens us to further options that are available to us.

Mental health has been described as the ability to move freely and flexibly in the world. Most mental health issues include an aspect of rigidity, in thinking, feeling, or behavior. For example, avoiding flying because of a phobia limits movement in the world, specifically the ability to go anyplace that requires air travel. Likewise, depression limits our ability to interact with others freely, feel the full range of emotions, and, because of the inhibiting effect on some aspects of cognition, consider a variety of choices in problem-solving. Functioning on autopilot means we may decrease flexibility by strengthening habitual thoughts, feelings, and behaviors through repetitive, automatic practice. Eventually, it takes a lot of effort to do or think about something in a new way. If you have ever broken or injured your dominant arm or hand, you know what I mean. Having to write, brush your teeth, or hold a fork with the weaker hand is almost like learning to do these things for the first time. Using the dominant hand is so automatic and well-practiced that you are rigid in your reliance on it.

Psychological flexibility is the by-product of engagement, and later in this chapter we will discuss the science behind this. Ultimately, the goal of practicing engagement is to move us out of a default position that limits our choices. With small moments of practice, engagement can become the new default.

"True life is lived when tiny changes occur."

—Leo Tolstoy

# THE REAL LIFE OF WALTER MITTY

You may recall Walter Mitty, the title character of James Thurber's classic short story (1939), who daydreams to escape the realities of his everyday world. In his fantastical fantasies, he is in control, powerful, dynamic, and adventurous. In his real life, he is ineffectual and unassertive. The theme of the dreamer who only dreams but does not "do" is one we find across cultures and time periods in literature and film. We relate to the courage and resilience required to take risks and "get in the game." In these stories, often an event or new insight pushes the dreamer to live more fully and to transform. Walter Mitty is a popular character because he is not exceptional or in possession of rare talents; he is a regular person like anyone you might meet on a daily basis. He is you and I.

Being engaged does not mean that you must give up daydreaming. Engagement requires that you focus intentionally on your real experience—including your sensations, thoughts, and feelings—in a nonevaluative way, and thus it is likely impossible to both be present and daydream at the same time. Yet daydreaming can be important as a rehearsal tool, such as when you practice in your head a difficult conversation before it occurs, or you imagine yourself completing an upcoming 5K race. Daydreaming can also be a coping tool when the present situation is difficult to endure. Daydreaming allows you to transcend your present circumstances and see possibilities. At the same time, daydreaming to avoid being in your daily life can pull you further from satisfaction and contentment when it shields you from self-awareness and impedes you from developing greater flexibility to act in your life. Engagement is about being in this moment in the here and now, rather than in the past or future.

# THE LIGHTS ARE ON BUT NOBODY'S HOME

Have you ever dragged yourself to work or another event or activity even though you were ill? Many feel that it is a badge of dedication to show up for the job even when sick, especially in the United States, where fortitude and overcoming adversity are highly valued. Physically you may be sitting at your desk, but mentally you're home lying on the couch watching talk shows. Showing up literally, but not figuratively, is an example of disengagement that hinders work/life balance.

Our ability to function on autopilot can prompt us to come to work when ill or mentally unavailable. We believe that we will function well on autopilot; in reality, though, we are unable to adequately perform our job duties. The disengagement we experience when we attempt to complete tasks while not fully able or invested is called *presenteeism*. Aronsson, Gustaffason, & Dallner (2000) define presenteeism as "people, despite complaints and ill health that should prompt rest and absence from work, still turning up at their jobs" (p. 503). Beyond acute and chronic illness, other episodic or chronic health conditions that contribute to presenteeism include migraines, arthritis and other chronic pain, asthma and seasonal allergies, and gastrointestinal issues (Hemp, 2004). Additionally, health risks, such as level of physical activity and body weight, have been shown to be related to presenteeism as well (Schultz & Edington, 2007). Lack of physical well-being is not the only reason that we may experience presenteeism. More recently, psychological health concerns, such as depression, have been incorporated into our understanding of presenteeism (Quazi, 2013). We may say that we occasionally need a "mental health day," but how many of us actually take one?

Presenteeism can be prompted by external pressures, including organizational culture, as well as the unique pressures created by the recent economic environment. Concerns about job security may lead employees to show up even when they are not performing at their best, and especially for those employees who are at risk for losing pay if they stay home (Widera, Chang, & Chen, 2010). In addition, internal pressures, such as perfectionism, self-criticism, a reluctance to disappoint others, or a need to be needed, are often the culprits behind presenteeism. We may struggle to say "no" and set boundaries (Aronsson & Gustafsson, 2005) in our daily lives both in and outside of work. Interestingly, helping professionals, such as health care professionals and educators, have the highest rates of coming to work while sick, despite typically working with the populations most vulnerable to the effects of contagious illnesses (Aronsson, Gustafsson, & Dallner, 2000). Of course, sometimes we simply have to care for sick children or other family members, or we become distracted by life events outside of work that then affect our attentiveness at work.

Engagement allows us both to understand our motives for our choices and to make better decisions about health and wellness. When we feel obligated to be present, engagement allows us to observe and understand these feelings of responsibility. By increasing awareness of the rationale for presenteeism, we learn more about our fundamental needs and motivators, and thus can be more present in our choices.

The relationship between stress and presenteeism is also discussed in Chapter 3.

# Presence on the Path to Balance

Mindfulness and flow are the two sides of the coin that represents engagement; they are two forms of here-and-now presence. Whereas mindfulness refers to increased self-awareness and focused consciousness in a moment, flow is about complete absorption in a task such that consciousness is transcended. Both are important tools for achieving balance, and we will explore how integrating mindfulness and flow into your life can enrich your sense of well-being and balance.

Typically when we work toward greater work/life balance, we focus on the things we have to do and on evening the scoreboard between time and effort in our professional and personal lives. We might calculate the time we spend in various activities to determine how we can simplify or delegate; alternatively, we might prioritize and focus on what can be achieved in the time we have. In either case, we attempt to minimize the amount of time we spend in unimportant tasks. Inevitably we find that there is simply not enough time to accomplish what is on our lists.

Engagement instead suggests that presence is the path to balance. Being more fully in the moment creates an experience of balance that does not involve a scorecard or counting time. Mindfulness and flow enable you to more fully experience your life so that you don't feel that time is wasted, you become less likely to feel burned out, and you achieve greater continuity among various facets of your life. The engaged you is always you, and you no longer feel like you are constantly changing hats to meet the demands of various roles in your life.

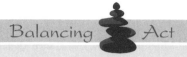

## MINDFUL ATTITUDES: THE BEGINNER'S MIND

Instead of going into the toy box, my son's playthings can remain on the dining room floor indefinitely. Eventually I don't see them anymore. They become part of the known landscape, and I instinctively lift my feet to avoid stepping on military guys and LEGOs without even thinking to pick them up. I lose awareness that the toys are spread on the floor because I expect them to be there. However, after cleaning the entire house for hours, I do notice the first time something winds up on the dining room floor. Eventually, I fall into the same ignoring pattern, but initially the novelty catches my eye.

Mindfulness practitioners aim to view experiences in life as if for the first time, with curiosity and openness. The Beginner's Mind enables you to view your daily life from a new angle and with a new awareness. Watching a child experience something for the first time can bring great joy and satisfaction, and when you see through a child's eyes, you use the Beginner's Mind.

Choose a moment in your day to practice viewing your world as through the eyes of a child. For example, when you get in the car to drive to work, imagine you have never seen or experienced a car. Notice the workings of the car, how it feels, how it sounds, how it smells. Notice the controls and their responses to your movements, and consider the ingenuity of the working machinery. In this moment, you will be practicing the Beginner's Mind, a foundational attitude in mindfulness.

# UNDERSTANDING MINDFULNESS

Mindfulness refers to intentionally focusing your attention in a non-judgmental and sustained fashion, thereby enhancing self-awareness in your life (Kabat-Zinn, 2012). The concept comes from Buddhism, where mindfulness is practiced formally, such as through regular meditation, and informally, in small moments throughout the day. Through mindfulness, you can experience your actions as choices and achieve a greater feeling of calm and control in your life, rather than experiencing your life as if it is going on around you without your direction.

The science behind mindfulness is well established. Mindfulness practice, training, and interventions, such as Mindfulness-Based Stress Reduction (MBSR) and Mindfulness-Based Cognitive Therapy (MBCT), have been associated with better immune functioning (Davidson et al., 2003); reduction in symptoms of anxiety disorders (Kabat-Zinn et al., 1992) and major depression (Galante, Iribarren, & Pearce, 2012); and improvement in psychosocial functioning associated with chronic somatic illness, such as cancer (Bohlmeijer, Prenger, Taal, & Cuijpers, 2010; Ledesma & Kumano, 2009); management of binge or overeating behavior (Kristeller & Wolever, 2011); decreased distress related to daily stress and hassles (Williams, Kolar, Reger, & Pearson, 2001); and reduced work-related burnout and stress (Flook, Goldberg, Pinker, Bonus, & Davidson, 2013; Goodman & Schorling, 2012).

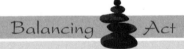

Balancing Act

## PRACTICING MINDFULNESS: MINDFUL EATING

A typical exercise for those beginning to practice mindfulness is to mindfully eat a raisin (Stahl & Goldstein, 2010). The purpose of the exercise is to be intentional in eating, to attend to the eating experience, and to curb self-criticism or judgment.

Prepare to eat the raisin by turning off all distractions, such as your phone, computer, television, and so on. You may substitute any food if you do not enjoy raisins or if a raisin is unavailable. Approach the raisin with the Beginner's Mind, as if you are a child who has never seen a raisin or you are from a place where raisins do not exist. Use all of your senses to experience the raisin. If you begin to have thoughts enter your mind, such as thinking the exercise is not worthwhile or boring, simply acknowledge the thoughts and return your awareness to the raisin.

Consider the raisin's physical traits. Notice the texture, the wrinkles, the weight, and the feel of the raisin. Do you notice that it is sticky or squishy? Notice the fine details on the skin of the raisin. Now smell the raisin, and breathe in its odor. Close your eyes if that is helpful to you. Listen to the raisin. Does it make a sound if you shake it or press on it? Notice your body as you bring the raisin to your mouth, and notice any sensations as you anticipate tasting the raisin. When the raisin is in your mouth, first notice how it feels to have the raisin in your mouth before you bite it. Now the taste: Is it sweet, slightly sour, or bitter? How does the raisin feel in your mouth and on your teeth? How does it feel when you bite into it and when you chew it? Notice the experience of swallowing the raisin and feeling it going into your digestive system.

Last, commend yourself for your willingness and effort to try this exercise.

*Adapted from* Mindfulness for Beginners *(Kabat-Zinn, 2012)*

## MANAGING STRESS IS LIKE DRIVING A CAR

When we experience stress or anxiety, the body, and specifically the autonomic nervous system (ANS), reacts as if we are in danger. The ANS is responsible for regulating involuntary body functions, such as digestion, respiration, and other organ functioning, and this system works in the background of our daily activities without our conscious awareness (Blechert, Grossman, Lajtman, & Wilhelm, 2007).

The sympathetic nervous system (SNS) is a subsystem of the ANS that readies us for addressing a dangerous situation. It shuts down nonvital functions in an emergency, such as digestion and reproduction, and then mobilizes vital organs, such as the lungs and heart, so that we can be prepared for fight or flight. The SNS is balanced by another ANS subsystem, the parasympathetic nervous system (PNS), which oversees our autonomic functioning in a state of rest or relaxation.

We can compare the SNS to a car's gas pedal and the PNS to the brake (Stahl & Goldstein, 2010). When we are in a hurry, we might drive faster, and the SNS shifts into high gear. We feel agitated and impatient, and yell at slow drivers. Physiologically, our heart rate and respiration increase, we begin to sweat, our pupils dilate, and our muscles tense as if ready to defend against an attacker. When the SNS is engaged, even at a red light, we feel the keen tension of preparedness for action. We are on the edge of the seat, waiting for the light to change.

After we have made it out of heavy traffic and we are close to our destination, the PNS can take over. The brake engages, and we slow down. Our shoulders, legs, arms, and jaw relax; we sit more comfortably in the seat; our pupils return to normal; our heart rate and respiration slow; and we might even notice that we feel hungry because, in the rush, we forgot to eat breakfast.

We rely on both of these ANS subsystems for survival, and together they serve to balance our body's response to the experience of stress in our environment. Because the ANS is unable to tell the difference between being stuck in traffic and being chased by a wild animal in the jungle, our bodies react in a similar fashion to any situation that stimulates the SNS to get us prepared to respond. What differs is our interpretation of these situations. Sustained and ongoing stress keeps the body in a constant state of alert, which can lead to a host of problems, such as high blood pressure, a weakened immune system, anxiety, and digestive ailments (Stahl & Goldstein, 2010).

Although the exact mechanism is not fully understood, it is believed that balance between the acceleration of the SNS and the deceleration of the PNS is responsible, at least in part, for our vulnerability to stress (Moore, Brown, Money, & Bates, 2011; Siegel, 2009). For instance, having the SNS engaged consistently during what should be relaxed moments can put us in a continuous state of stress. Significantly anxious individuals sometimes report that they find it difficult to "turn off" stress and find themselves experiencing the physiological and emotional components of anxiety even when they recognize it as unnecessary. The setting or situation alone can trigger the SNS to accelerate out of habit. For those who experience constant stress and pressure at work, for example, the SNS can gear up simply when a person thinks about work.

One of my patients explained that she was so used to worrying about running late that she felt anxiety, agitation, increased heart rate, sweating, and increased respiration when she walked from place to place even when she would clearly arrive on time. She said that the anxiety and accompanying physiological experiences were automatic; she had felt them for so long that she began to feel them without noticing and without actual cause. She said that she could not remember what it felt like not to be stressed out or anxious. Mindfulness helped her to become more aware of these feelings and bodily sensations, to identify if they actually fit the situation at hand, and then to adjust her experience to better fit the circumstances.

In *The Mindful Brain* (2007), Daniel Siegel suggests that mindfulness practice enables us to better balance the SNS and the PNS to bring ourselves back to a relaxation state when we gain awareness of a stress reaction. Mindfulness can also change the brain. Specifically, research supports that practicing mindfulness can thicken the cortex in brain regions related to learning, self-awareness, and emotional intelligence (Holzel et al., 2011). Regular mindfulness practice increases neural plasticity, or flexibility in brain functions (Siegel, 2009), thereby enabling us to practice new patterns of attending and sensing, change our patterns of thinking, feeling, and behaving, and increase our ability to regulate emotion (Lazar et al., 2005; Siegel, 2009).

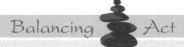

Balancing Act

## MINDFUL ATTITUDES: NONSTRIVING AND SELF-COMPASSION

I once provided marital therapy for a couple in which both husband and wife struggled with disappointment. At first, it appeared that their discontent was directed outward, toward ineffective healthcare providers, teachers, and employees, and inadequate parents, friends, and siblings. They often focused on what was missing or not going well in their lives, and, more specifically, what was not living up to their expectations. Their dissatisfaction inevitably was focused on each other, leading to blame, resentment, and disrespect.

In trying to find language to help them talk about their experiences, I explained that they were "living in the gap," meaning living in the space between their beliefs about what life should be like and what life was really like. This space left them in limbo, in between worlds, with neither grounding nor achievable aspirations. In the gap, they were stuck in feelings of pessimism, entitlement, and loss.

*continues*

*continued*

In fact, after some reflection, we realized that this couple's discontent was really a result of their own feelings of inadequacy. They felt vulnerable, incompetent, and not good enough at parenting, earning money, making friends, and generally the business of being adults. For every experience in their lives they filled out a mental evaluation form, and they were failing miserably. What they truly wished was for someone to help them, to show them how to manage their lives, but they felt so helpless that no helper could be up to the task, leaving them feeling let down by the world.

Because this couple, living in the gap, found it impossible to find a competent and trustworthy babysitter, I agreed to hold a few therapy sessions via video-conferencing in order to work toward their hiring a sitter. One evening, I noticed in the background on the wall of the husband's home office, a motivational poster. You know the kind of poster I mean. It had SUCCESS in big letters across the top, and a picture of a beautiful, strong whale cresting in a huge, foamy ocean.

Because they both had a good sense of humor, I asked them to create a new poster to hang on top of the SUCCESS poster with the title GOOD ENOUGH. I asked them to cover the cresting whale with photos of themselves doing everyday things. Although they found this homework exercise comical, they also noticed the irony in their struggle to come up with the absolute best way to complete the new poster.

Nonstriving is a mindful attitude that encourages us to focus on what is true rather than what we wish were true. The attitude of self-compassion means a nonjudgmental, noncritical, and accepting approach. It is healthy to set goals and to challenge ourselves to achieve them; in fact, doing so is a key element in experiencing contentment, as we cover later in this chapter in the discussion of flow. Yet, living in the gap is instead a fantasy that leads to helplessness and dissatisfaction. In mindfulness practice, we "strive" to be nonstriving, focused not on achieving any specific outcome, but rather engaging ourselves in a kind, compassionate, and nonjudgmental way. There is no successful or unsuccessful mindfulness practice, no effective or ineffective practitioner, only you in your real life.

## Practicing Mindfulness

Mindfulness practice can be formal, such as through mindfulness meditation, or informal, such as eating your lunch or folding the laundry mindfully. Informal mindfulness practice occurs in your daily activities by focusing on intention, attention, and attitude, the building blocks of mindful being (Shapiro, Carlson, Astin, & Freeman, 2006). Intending to be mindful, focusing attention toward self-awareness, and practicing mindful attitudes—such as the Beginner's Mind, Nonstriving, and Self-Compassion—are the three fundamental steps in daily mindfulness.

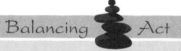

Balancing Act

### Everyday Mindfulness

Try bringing intention, attention, and mindful attitudes to these everyday moments:

- **Morning routine:** While showering or brushing your teeth, notice if you are ruminating or planning, and bring your focus back to the experience. Notice the smells, sensations, and sounds.

- **Walking:** Notice your thoughts and body positioning. Move your shoulder blades back and relax your shoulders. Refocus on your body and notice your breathing, your feet and legs, and the experience of movement.

- **Interacting with others:** Notice if you are thinking about what you want to say next, and refocus on what the other person is saying. Experience their verbal and nonverbal cues and notice yourself listening to them.

- **Household chores:** Washing dishes, vacuuming, and other household activities are typical times when we are not mindful. While doing these tasks, notice what you are thinking and feeling, and focus on being present and fully experiencing the task at hand.

- **Mindful check-in:** Use a phone or tablet app or notification to remind yourself to be mindful. For 60 seconds, notice yourself. What is your mood? How does your body feel? Are you present and engaged in what you are doing? Is your mind wandering? What are you thinking about? Return to your activity with greater presence.

Meditation is one tool for formal mindfulness practice. Meditation can last for 5 minutes each day or can be built up to longer periods. Breathing, body awareness, posture, refocusing wandering thoughts, and attending to sensations and feelings are key aspects of any mindfulness meditation practice. In addition, yoga can be used as an instrument for formal mindful practice. Some experimentation will aid you in discovering what meditation is your best fit. At the end of this chapter are resources for accessing guided meditations.

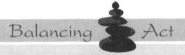

Balancing Act

## FIVE-MINUTE MEDITATION

Five minutes of meditation is enough for many to feel ready to face the day with presence and engagement. This meditation can be particularly grounding as you leave your home life to enter the workplace, such as in the morning, or when you first return home. Some find it helpful during a lunch break to reinvigorate for the rest of the day. It can aid you as a daily reminder to be present or in transitioning between environments with distinct demands.

Find a place to sit or lie down comfortably. Rest your hands at your sides or in another comfortable and relaxed position. If you find that you fall asleep while lying down during this exercise then try sitting instead. Close your eyes if you want. Offer congratulations to yourself for this time you have set aside to practice.

Notice your breathing. Notice the air flowing into your body, moving down your throat and filling your lungs or diaphragm. Notice the breath leaving your body. It may feel cool entering, and warmer as it leaves. Notice the rhythm of your breath, and how your chest expands and falls as the breath enters and leaves. How does your breathing sound? What are the sensations?

Your mind will likely wander. Acknowledge the thought or feeling and refocus on your breathing. Do not judge the thought, such as, "Stop thinking and focus," or "I'm wasting time." Simply acknowledge the thought, and let it be. Then return to your breathing. Just notice your natural breathing. Tell yourself that you are present in this moment, and that you have nowhere else to be in this moment. You may want to set a reminder bell on your phone, clock, or computer to let you know when the 5-minute practice time has passed.

Congratulate yourself on your practice, and acknowledge the self-caring and self-compassion you expressed in giving yourself this time to practice.

*Adapted from* A Mindfulness-Based Stress Reduction Workbook *(Stahl & Goldstein, 2010)*

"Happiness is absorption."

—T.E. Lawrence

## FLOW

Now it's time to explore the other side of the engagement coin, specifically flow. Mindfulness increases self-awareness, but *flow* is achieved through losing yourself in an absorbing task. Flow is a second path to engagement, in which acute self-awareness is not only impossible, but in fact a hindrance.

The concept of flow originated from Mihaly Csikszentmihalyi's work on understanding what makes people happy (Csikszentmihalyi, 1990). He and his colleagues around the globe asked people to wear a specially developed pager. When prompted during the day by the pager, the people would record what they were doing and feeling (Csikszentmihalyi, 1990). Csikszentmihalyi's research team discovered that activities associated with happy feelings ranged widely from mountain climbing to mowing the lawn. Despite this variety, the description of the experience was similar among these "happy" activities. People felt happy in what are called "flow" activities.

Interestingly, we are acutely aware when we are unhappy or depressed, but when we are happy, we typically do not stop to notice it; instead, we are engaged in the moment (Kral & Idlout, 2012). Like mindfulness, flow involves gaining control over consciousness, increasing psychological flexibility, and increasing here-and-now engagement. As with mindfulness, self-consciousness disappears in flow. We forget what is going on around us as we focus on the present.

## *Elements of Flow*

Flow occurs in activities in which we are fully focused and engaged, concentrating, and somewhat challenged. Just kicking back and relaxing is not typically considered a flow activity because it does not require concentration or focus, although many report that they do feel relaxed during flow activities. According to Csikszentmihalyi, flow is "a state in which people are so involved in an activity that nothing else seems to matter; the experience itself is so enjoyable that people will do it even at great cost, for the sheer sake of doing it" (Csikszentmihalyi, 1990, p. 4).

We must be able to concentrate to experience flow. For many, spending time with or caring for children is a flow experience. Building with LEGOs or completing an art project with a child may be a flow experience, but working on your own project while distracted by a child is unlikely to bring flow. At work, distractions often interrupt flow experiences. If you have ever felt that you need to shut the office door or turn off email alerts in order to get things done, then you know what I mean.

Flow requires clear goals and instant feedback. Many report housecleaning to be a flow experience. The goal is very clear, and we instantly know if we missed a spot. Reading a book also fits the criteria. Reading is more about the experience of the book than it is about the achievement of reaching the end. Yet, when reading a good mystery, I often find myself checking to see how many pages are left until I reach the surprise ending. With nonfiction in particular, new insight can be our goal, and as we read, our learning serves as instant feedback.

Our sense of time shifts in flow. We may feel as if time has flown by. Anyone who has wiled the hours away playing Angry Birds or binge-watched an entire season of a television show in one sitting knows what this is about. Actually, television presents an interesting paradox when viewed through the lens of flow. Watching television is typically considered a passive activity. Watching the 100th rerun of a show we do not particularly enjoy just to pass the time actually tends to make us unhappy and dissatisfied with life. On the other hand, an engaging and challenging show can provide a flow experience. Shows such as *Lost*, in which the viewer struggles to piece together what the action means, or programs that engage the viewer in taking a new perspective or gaining new insight can certainly be experienced as flow.

With mindfulness, we may experience our everyday worries and thoughts, but we attempt to refocus on the present moment. In flow, we forget our troubles and we forget ourselves; as Csikszentmihalyi says, "concern for the self disappears, yet paradoxically the sense of self emerges stronger after the flow experience" (1990, p. 49). Because flow activities can be challenging, we may come away with a sense of accomplishment that enables us to feel stronger and more capable. In fact, we rely on our skill level to provide a sense of control that may not actually exist. Someone without adequate skill might feel overwhelmed and out of control in activities such as riding a motorcycle or skiing, but the person with sufficient skill will instead experience flow. Flow activities require that we have the skill to actually complete the task, and the balance or "sweet spot" between skill and challenge is the key (Jackson & Eklund, 2012). If we are not challenged by a task, we experience boredom or apathy. If we are too challenged, we feel frustration or anxiety.

## Flow in Balance

Unlike mindfulness, flow experiences typically have a goal. Yet, we participate in flow activities for their own sake, not for the sake of the accomplishment. For example, we may play soccer with the goal of winning the game; however, flow comes not from the winning, but from the playing. Flow can come from either activities of obligation or choice.

So how does flow relate to balance? Flow can be found in any setting, and many report flow in their work lives, even in tasks that appear routine or repetitive. In fact, those who experience the greatest job satisfaction and commitment tend to find flow at work (Maeran & Cangiano, 2013). If you have ever felt that you would do your job for free, you likely experience flow at work. When we feel the weight of obligation in our work lives, including boredom and apathy, we likely feel that we are out of balance.

Many organizations have turned to flow research to promote greater creativity and productivity in their employees. Because flow occurs at the sweet spot between challenge and skill, strategies include increasing challenge or creating opportunities for employees to develop and use different skills (Maymin, 2011). On mundane tasks, we can even create our own milestone challenges or make a game out of it. For example, when I have to stuff envelopes, I aim to see how many I can finish in 1 minute.

On the other hand, workplace stress may be due in part to the level of challenge overwhelming our skills, which often means not that we lack the skills for any one task but rather that our overall workload is simply too great to manage effectively. Unfortunately, we may fail to ask for help because we fear being perceived as unskilled or as complainers. Especially in the current economic climate, many of us are doing the jobs of two or more people as the organizations we work for tighten their belts. Prioritizing becomes critical in these instances, and where possible, so does delegation or asking for help or resources (Maymin, 2011). Requests for additional training or skill development may be better received than asking for additional hands that may simply be unavailable. Teaming up with a coworker with different but complementary skills to contribute to each other's projects is a strategy that can decrease work stress. Recently a research project required me to conduct statistical analyses well out of my skill level. I teamed up with a colleague who is a great statistician, but who is not as skilled in applying the findings to the real world. He figures out the "what," and I figure out the "why." It has been a fruitful partnership, and we now collaborate on multiple projects, decreasing both of our stress levels.

Finding opportunities for flow can increase our experience of well-being and happiness at work and in our lives and enhance our ability to achieve balance. Ongoing learning and engagement in which we balance skill and challenge can enable us to experience flow every day. Engaging in this way means we are flying, but we are not on autopilot.

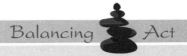

Balancing Act

## ASSESSING FLOW

Consider if you are adequately challenged at work. Does your job hit the "sweet spot" in balancing skill and challenge? What tasks or activities provide you with flow at work? When do you feel a sense of obligation in your job? Are there ways in which you can incorporate elements of flow into this task?

## EXERCISE

Make a list with two columns, one including the work experiences that cause you stress, and the other those that lead to boredom. For the items in the stress column, generate strategies for how you can develop skills, prioritize, and let things go, or collaborate with coworkers to decrease stress. Alternatively, for the items in the boredom column, generate strategies for how you can increase your level of challenge or complete the tasks in a way such that you use less perfected skills.

Now, let's see how you balance flow at work and in your life. Make another list with two columns: one column for flow activities in your life and the other for flow activities at work. Life flow can include daily tasks, such as cleaning or cooking; hobbies, such as sports, music, hiking, writing, or video games; interpersonal activities, such as socializing, entertaining, or playing; or religious or spiritual experiences. The work list can include any flow tasks, simple to highly complex. Notice where you experience more flow—at work or in life. If you only find flow at work, you may run the risk of workaholism. If you only find flow at home, you may experience deep dissatisfaction with your job. Or are your lists fairly even? Do you find opportunities for flow both at work and in your life? If you experience boredom and apathy in your nonwork life, are there ways that you can implement the strategies of increasing challenge or using less-developed skills? And if you experience stress and anxiety in your daily life, are there ways that you can increase skill, prioritize, let go, or collaborate?

# Small Steps on the Path to Engagement

Turning off autopilot and experiencing greater presence in your daily life can reduce stress and burnout, promote balance, and enhance creativity and productivity. Engagement happens both by noticing and not noticing oneself—like two sides of a coin—through mindfulness and flow.

Practicing mindfulness, intention, attention, and mindful attitude can bring about physiological changes that increase psychological flexibility. Self-awareness allows you to make better choices in the moment rather than relying on habit, the old default position. Practicing one mindful moment each day is a great start.

On the other hand, flow allows you to stop noticing yourself and to experience full immersion in a task that is challenging but attainable. Flow activities boost our sense of competence and make us feel happier, more alive, and stronger. Like mindfulness practice, flow can be experienced in small moments rather than require a radical shift. Adjusting your skill or challenge level can bring flow to an everyday task.

Mindfulness and flow are the paths to presence, and will enable you to shift your default position to being in the moment, and ultimately, in your life.

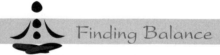

## Resources for Mindfulness and Flow

**Mindfulness**

- Stahl, B. & Goldstein, E. (2010). *A mindfulness-based stress reduction workbook*. Oakland, CA: New Harbinger. Provides meditation lessons with increasing skill, including a CD with guided meditations.

- UCLA Mindful Awareness Research Center (http://marc. ucla.edu/body.cfm?id=22). Free guided meditations of varying lengths.

- Mindfulness Daily app by Inward (iOS). Reminders and trackers for daily mindful moments, audio lesson, relaxation practice, meditation, and a mindfulness log.

- Headspace app (iOS and Android). Daily meditations and programs focused specifically on stress, eating, and sleep; reminders; a tracking log; and a dashboard to see your overall progress.

- Mindfulness Meditation app (iOS and Android). Beginning-level app that includes an 8-week, formal meditation program with 5- to 40-minute guided meditations.

- Breathe2Relax app (iOS and Android). Focuses on various types of breathing and increasing your control of your breathing in distinct emotional states.

**Flow**

- Csikszentmihalyi, M. (1998). *Finding flow: The psychology of engagement with everyday life.* New York: Basic Books. Csikszentmihalyi explains his research on happiness and flow activities, with an emphasis on helping you to apply his findings to increase flow in your daily life.

- Kotler, S. (2014). *The rise of superman: Decoding the science of ultimate human performance.* New York: New Harvest. Kotler uses examples from extreme professional sports to demonstrate how flow can improve performance and increase well-being for you and me.

# Reflections

- Experience presence and balance in your life through mindfulness and flow.

- Practice a mindful moment each day during your morning routine, a chore, or as you eat a snack.

- Approach the mindful task with the Beginner's Mind, Non-striving, and Self-Compassion.

- Consider whether you experience flow both at work and in your life.

- Find the "sweet spot" between stress and boredom by increasing challenge, using less-developed skills, partnering with others, prioritizing, or participating in ongoing learning.

# References

Aronsson, G., & Gustafsson, K. (2005). Sickness presenteeism: Prevalence, attendance-pressure factors and an outline of a model for research. *Journal of Occupational Environmental Medicine, 47*(9), 958-966.

Aronsson, G., Gustafsson, K., & Dallner, M. (2000). Sick but yet at work: An empirical study of sickness presenteeism. *Journal of Epidemiology and Community Health, 54*(7), 502-509.

Blechert, M. J., Grossman, P., Lajtman, M., & Wilhelm, F. H. (2007). Autonomic and respiratory characteristics of posttraumatic stress disorder and panic disorder. *Psychosomatic Medicine, 69*(9), 935-943.

Bohlmeijer, E., Prenger, R., Taal, E., & Cuijpers, P. (2010). The effects of mindfulness-based stress reduction therapy on mental health of adults with a chronic medical disease: A meta-analysis. *Journal of Psychosomatic Research, 68*(6), 539-544. doi: 10.1016/j.jpsychores.2009.10.005

Csikszentmihalyi, M. (1990). *Flow: The psychology of optimal experience*. New York: Harper & Row.

Davidson, R. J., Kabat-Zinn, J., Schumacher, J., Rosenkranz, M., Muller, D., Santorelli, S.,…Sheridan, J. (2003). Alterations in brain and immune function produced by mindfulness meditation. *Psychosomatic Medicine, 65*(4), 546-570. doi: 10.1097/01.PSY.0000077505.67574.E3

Duckworth, A. L., Steen, T. A., & Seligman, M. E. P. (2005). Positive psychology in clinical practice. *Annual Review of Clinical Psychology, 1*, 629-651.

Flook, L., Goldberg, S. B., Pinger, L., Bonus, K., & Davidson, R. J. (2013). Mindfulness for teachers: A pilot study to assess effects on stress, burnout, and teaching efficacy. *Mind, Brain, and Education, 7*(3), 182-195.

Galante, J., Iribarren, S. J., & Pearce, P. F. (2012). Effects of mindfulness-based cognitive therapy on mental disorders: A systematic review and meta-analysis of randomized controlled trials. *Journal of Research in Nursing, 18*(2), 133-155.

Goodman, M. J., & Schorling, J. B. (2012). A mindfulness course decreases burnout and improves well-being among healthcare providers. *International Journal of Psychiatry in Medicine, 43*(2), 119-128.

Hemp, P. (2004). Presenteeism: At work, but out of it. *Harvard Business Review, 82*(10), 49-58.

Holzel, B. K., Lazar, S., Gard, T., Schuman-Olivier, Z., Vago, D. R., & Ott, U. (2011). How does mindfulness meditation work? Proposing mechanisms of action from a conceptual and neural perspective. *Perspectives on Psychological Science, 6*(6), 537-559. doi: 10.1177/1745691611419671

Jackson, S., & Eklund, R. C. (2012). Flow. In G. Tenebaum, R. C. Eklund & A. Kamata, (Eds.), *Measurement in sport and exercise psychology* (pp. 349-357). Champaign, IL: Human Kinetics, US.

Kabat-Zinn, J. (2012). *Mindfulness for beginners.* Boulder, CO: Sounds True.

Kabat-Zinn, J., Massion, A. O., Kristeller, J., Peterson, L. G., Flecher, K. E., Pbert, L.,...Santorelli, S. F. (1992). Effectiveness of a meditation-based stress reduction program in the treatment of anxiety disorders. *American Journal of Psychiatry,* 14(9), 936-943.

Kral, M. & Idlout, L. (2012). It's all in the family: Wellbeing among Inuit in arctic Canada. In H. Selin & G. Davey (Eds.), *Happiness across cultures: Views of happiness and quality of life in non-Western cultures* (pp. 387-398). New York: Springer Science and Business Media.

Kristeller, J. L., & Wolever, R. Q. (2011). Mindfulness-based eating awareness training for treating binge eating disorder: The conceptual foundation. *Eating Disorders, 19*(1), 49-61. doi: 10.1080/10640266.2011.533605

Lazar, S. W., Kerr, C. E., Wasserman, R. H., Gray, J. R., Greve, D. N., Treadway, M. T.,... Fischl, B. (2005). Meditation experience is associated with increased cortical thickness. *Neuroreport, 16*(17), 1893-1897.

Ledesma, D., & Kumano, H. (2009). Mindfulness-based stress reduction and cancer: A meta-analysis. *Psychooncology, 18*(6), 571-579. doi: 10.1002/pon.1400

Maeran, R., & Cangiano, F. (2013). Flow experience and job characteristics: Analyzing the role of flow in job satisfaction. *TPM-Testing, Psychometrics, Methodology in Applied Psychology, 20*(1), 13-26.

Maymin, S. (2011). Flow at work: Three questions. PBS *This Emotional Life.* Retrieved from http://www.pbs.org/thisemotionallife/blogs/flow

Moore, M., Brown, D., Money, N., & Bates, M. (2011). Mind-body skills for regulating the autonomic nervous system, v.2. Defense Centers of Excellence for Psychological Health and Traumatic Brain Injury. Retrieved from http://www.dcoe.mil/content/Navigation/Documents/Mind-Body%20Skills%20for%20Regulating%20the%20Autonomic%20Nervous%20System.pdf

Quazi, H. (2013). *Presenteeism: The invisible cost to organizations.* New York: Palgrave MacMillan.

Schultz, A. B., & Edington, D. W. (2007). Employee health and presenteeism: A systematic review. *Journal of Occupational Rehabilitation, 17*(3), 547-579. doi: 10.1007/s10926-007-9096-x

Seligman, M. E. P. (1975). *Helplessness: On depression, development, and death.* San Francisco: W. H. Freeman.

Seligman, M. E. P., & Peterson, C. (2003). Positive clinical psychology. In L. G. Aspinwall & U. M. Staudinger, (Eds.), *A psychology of human strengths: Fundamental questions and future directions for a positive psychology* (pp. 305-317). Washington, DC: American Psychological Association.

Shapiro, S. L., Carlson, L., Astin, J., & Freedman, B. (2006). Mechanisms of mindfulness. *Journal of Clinical Psychology, 62*(3), 373-386.

Siegel, D. J. (2007). *The mindful brain: Reflection and attunement in the cultivation of well-being.* New York: Norton.

Siegel, D. J. (2009). Mindful awareness, mindsight, and neural integration. *The Humanistic Psychologist, 37*(2), 137-158.

Stahl, B., & Goldstein, E. (2010). A mindfulness-based stress reduction workbook. Oakland, CA: New Harbinger.

Thurber, J. (1939, March 18). The secret life of Walter Mitty. *The New Yorker*, 19-20.

Widera, E., Chang, A., & Chen, H. L. (2010). Presenteeism: A public health hazard. *Journal of General Internal Medicine, 25*(11), 1244-1247. doi: 10.1007/s11606-010-1422-x

Williams, K. A., Kolar, M. M., Reger, B. E., & Pearson, J. C. (2001). Evaluation of a wellness-based mindfulness stress reduction intervention: A controlled trial. *American Journal of Health Promotion, 15*(6), 422-432. doi: http://dx.doi.org/10.4278/0890-1171-15.6.422

> "In your thirst for knowledge, be sure not to drown in all the information."
>
> —Anthony J. D'Angelo

# 6

# PUTTING TECHNOLOGY IN ITS PLACE: THE EFFECT OF CONNECTIVITY AND SOCIAL MEDIA

*–Sharon M. Weinstein, MS, RN, CRNI, FACW, FAAN*

Information overload is not only possible; it is probable in today's work environment. Regardless of your role within the system, if you're feeling swamped, get help. Learning to let go of the "stuff" in your life is the first step toward avoiding information overload. The lines between your personal and public lives, your work and play, your friends and families may have blurred due to the social era in which we live. How do you draw the line between privacy and the need to know? Are you in danger due to overexposure to connectivity? How can you cope with information overload in a highly technical world? Do social media and connectivity prevent you from having a life in balance?

Does technology help or is it another form of information overload? Do you really need to know every detail, be part of every meeting, or read every piece of information you come across? Technology should support and enable your home and business processes, not dictate how your life is run. It's up to you to control how you use technology, and not let the technology control you. This chapter takes a look at the benefits of technology, the problems that technology can cause you, and how you can balance your use of it in your life.

# TECHNOLOGY CAN BE TOO MUCH OF A GOOD THING

Life is bound to throw you a few curveballs. Chances are they may relate to technology. What do you do when the unexpected comes crashing into your world? Do your palms sweat? Does your heart skip a beat? Your system crashed, and you think, "How did this happen?"

Technology has simplified and complicated our lives. From electronic records to text messaging, our lives have changed and can sometimes seem to be controlled by bits and bytes. In an instant, we can send an email message telling everyone on the "To" list the exact same thing at the exact same time. (Don't we all know someone who has clicked Send on a "Reply All" email message and instantly regretted it?) Before, we could send one postal letter at a time or make one phone call at a time. We took the time to proofread and double-check our work or words. In addition to using email, we can also IM (instant message), text, tweet, blog, write on our or someone else's Facebook walls, tag (photos), and receive endless RSS (Rich Site Summary) feeds. In sum, we have far more contact with far more people and information on a daily basis than ever before in human history. This can create unnecessary stress in our lives when we try to keep up with everything. But it is okay to not keep up with everything!

*"I think it's very important to get more women into computing. My slogan is: Computing is too important to be left to men."*

—Karen Sparck Jones

# FROM MAC TO REALITY

Thirty years ago, Apple introduced the Macintosh computer with the promise to put the creative power of technology in everyone's hands. It launched a generation of innovators who continue to change the world (Apple, 2014).

Over the course of 30 years, Apple introduced a computer that transformed our lives and made everyone want to own a computer. The first "box" computer was rather primitive by today's standards. It required lots of codes to enable it to print to roller paper, and it was challenging to use. I have many colleagues whose kids taught them to type, print, and save on an Apple. And, along came electronic music in 1985 when electro-acoustic composer Jon Appleton created one of the first digital music studios in the world, and it was built around the Macintosh XL.

In 1987, Theodore Gray used a Macintosh to create a science- and math-based computer program aimed at organizing data. Technology at its finest! This development was followed by the ability to integrate a digital or display font that anyone could use, creating new opportunities for artists and storytellers to use programs like Adobe's Illustrator to generate exciting documents.

Then in 1989 along came Photoshop—a program that I still have not mastered. The world of manipulation of images had begun. The early 1990s brought video games to the forefront, followed by soundtrack music, graphic novels, and digital magazines like *Rolling Stone*. Good things blossom—and 30 years has been good for Apple and its competitors. They have transformed communication, education, science, and even surgery.

There is little doubt that yesterday's technology, like a Sony Walkman, looks silly to today's children, and much of today's technology will appear silly to the next generation. Think about it: CDs, DVDs, and minidiscs are being replaced. Do you recall carrying a pager at one time during your career? Maps have given way to GPS navigation systems. I recall when our grandson was a toddler and his parents were actively discussing which way to go to get to the park. Seated in his car seat in the back of the car, he said, "You need a map; Dora has a map." Of course, if the popular TV character could find her way with a map, his parents should be able to do the same. Now, they use a GPS!

Do you recall dial-up Internet access and collections of media, cords, and cables? How did we manage without email and text messaging? But those tools may be our downfall!

# PRIVACY OR THE NEED TO KNOW

We value our privacy; think about the party lines of long ago when a call could be interrupted because a neighbor needed to speak to a family member or friend. It was no party! (For those who do not know what a party line is, ask your parents or grandparents to tell you.)

Cybercrime is a threat; we have seen the results of cybercrime in our own lifetimes through breaches in online retailers' security as well as with social media. Should surveillance by government be permitted? Computer and network intrusions, along with identity theft, are valid concerns. Credit card consumer fraud, online shopping fraud, and investment fraud—these and more are signs of the times. Do we have too many tools at our disposal? How do we balance our own privacy against our need to know (Miller, 2011)?

*"Lo! Men have become the tools of their tools."*
*—Henry David Thoreau*

# CONNECTIVITY

Being connected is a good thing; now that we have experienced it, we demand it. We want more and more access. We want smart schools with Wi-Fi everywhere. We are facing a serious threat to our health, and with time, being always connected will challenge our health and our future. It is no secret that the public is increasingly concerned about exposure to Wi-Fi, cell masts, smart meters, and more (Copes, 2011; Dean, Rea, Smith, & Barrier, n.d.).

Is connectivity unsafe for students, and is it in your child's school or in your own home? The effect on students' health is real and is manifested as headaches, eye strain, the sensation that something is irritating the eyes, dizziness, and increased heart rate. Children who live in homes with no Wi-Fi (or where it is turned off) experience the symptoms at school but find they disappear when they gets home! Cellular phones present similar challenges (Aldad, Gan, Gao, & Taylor, 2012).

## IMPACT ON HEALTH

Radiation from cell phones is too weak to heat biological tissue or break chemical bonds in cells, but the radio waves the phones emit may still change cell behavior. Scientists exposed 10 female volunteers to radiation at 900 megahertz from GSM phones to simulate an hour-long phone call.

They screened 580 different proteins in their skin cells and found that the numbers of two proteins were altered in all of the volunteers: one protein increased by 89%, the other decreased by 32%.

They demonstrated that even without heating, molecular level changes take place in response to exposure to cell phone frequency electromagnetic radiation. So what is the physiological significance of these changes in proteins? So far, no one knows for sure. However, I firmly believe that dismissing it as inconsequential would be a serious mistake, especially in light of the data available that suggests a variety of long-term health risks (Dean et al., n.d.).

## WHAT CAUSES THE BIOLOGICAL DAMAGE?

Let me be clear. Most of the danger from most land-based portable phones, cell phones, and Wi-Fi routers is not from the thermal damage produced by these devices. Unless you have massive exposures like you might expect in a microwave oven, these thermal effects are insignificant. Experts believe the biological damage comes both from the modulated signals that are carried *on* the carrier microwave and the carrier wave itself. However, they do their damage by two entirely different mechanisms. These modulated information-carrying radio waves resonate in biological frequencies of a few to a few hundred cycles per second and can stimulate your cellular receptors, thus causing a whole cascade of pathological consequences that can culminate in fatigue, anxiety, and, ultimately, cancers. Funk, Monsees, and Ozkucur noted many advances in our understanding of electromagnetic fields (2009). Volkow and associates (2011) stated that 50-minute cell phone exposure was associated with increased brain glucose metabolism in the region closest to the antenna.

This is a *major* problem because in the last few years we have had an exponential increase in exposure to these waves. It took from 1984 to 2004 to reach the first billion cell phones; the second billion took just 18 months; the third billion took only 9 months; and the fourth billion just 6 months.

These numbers do not factor in any of your exposure to Wi-Fi routers, which are now pervasive. Because there is a lag time of 5 to 20 years before many of the effects become clinically apparent, now is the time to act before you or your family suffer the damage.

## YOU MAY ALREADY SUFFER THE ILL EFFECTS

Numerous studies claim there is no biological impact of radio frequency (RF) radiation within the cell phone range. Additionally, researchers in different countries are finding equally disturbing results that point to far greater health implications than anyone is ready for. The U.S. Food and Drug Administration (2012) acknowledges the concerns and the unknowns, such as the effect of increased temperature from electromagnetic energy. According to Fathi and Farahzadi (2014), available data do not suggest any immediate cause for concern of an impending threat to the health of the population from acute or short-term exposure to low level RF radiation.

> For ongoing discussions of this important topic, you can check out http://www.ihfglobal.com/emf_education.html.

Unfortunately, most people fail to correlate common symptoms and health problems to their exposure to cell phones and other radio frequencies, perhaps because these conditions can so easily be attributed to other causes as well.

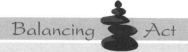

Balancing Act

## AILMENTS LINKED TO CELL PHONE RADIO WAVES

Do you suffer from any of these common illnesses and ailments, which have all been scientifically linked to cell phone information-carrying radio waves?

- Alzheimer's, senility, and dementia
- Parkinson's
- Autism
- Fatigue
- Headaches
- Sleep disruptions
- Altered memory function, poor concentration, and spatial awareness

Although cancer and brain tumors are most often cited as the potential health risks from cell phone radiation, as you can see, cancer is not the only, or the most common, danger that you and your children face.

## Is Your Headset Making Matters Worse?

For some time, the standard recommendation to reduce your radiation exposure was to use a headset. However newer investigations and the emergence of wireless earpieces (such as Bluetooth) turn this idea upside down. These headsets may actually intensify your exposure to harmful radiation because the headset itself acts as an antenna, which is inserted directly into your ear canal (Centers for Disease Control and Prevention [CDC], 2013).

Testing has indicated that your cell phone headset may actually raise the amount of radiation emitted by more than 300%! It's vital that you know the pros and cons of cell phone headsets, especially now that laws requiring "hands-free" cell phone use while driving are going into effect all over the United States.

Headsets are an ideal solution only if they are used with filters to stop the headset wire from acting as an effective antenna. One solution is an air tube headset. These conduct sound but prevent any radiation from traveling up the wire to your brain. The cord is about 3 feet long and uses a clear plastic tube to carry the sound to your ear. There are no electronics involved.

# More Safety Tips to Limit Your Exposure

To date, there are few alternatives to ensure complete safety, but there are some common sense recommendations:

1. Limit the amount of time you spend on the phone.

2. Limit your exposure to Wi-Fi routers. Find out where they are located in your work environment and stay away from them.

3. If you have any land-based (noncellular) portable phones, do *not* use anything other than the 900 MHz phones as the Gigahertz phones stay on continuously, blasting you with information-carrying radio waves 24/7.

4. Use the speakerphone instead of putting the phone to your ear; this is probably one of the single most important steps you can take other than not using your cell phone.

5. Use a wired headset to limit your exposure to the cell phone—ideally, an air tube headset that conducts sound but prevents any radiation from traveling up the wire to your brain. Also make sure the wire is shielded, which prevents the wire from acting as an antenna that could attract more information-carrying radio waves directly to your brain.

6. Limit calls inside buildings.

7. Use the phone in open spaces as often as possible.

8. Limit use by children and preadolescents.

# LONG-TERM EFFECTS

There are no safe levels of radiation. The mass rollout of Wi-Fi over the past decade has been phenomenal; Wi-Fi has become integrated in all facets of our society and our personal lives. Yet few have asked the most important of all questions: Is it safe? At what levels does ever increasing Wi-Fi become dangerous to human health? Can it, or is it, affecting our electronic bodies, our well-being, and our abilities to think? To what degree, if any, do invisible radio and microwave frequencies begin to affect our own DNA structures?

Over the past few years, and secretly for decades, scientific and medical evidence has shown conclusively that the low frequency pulsed radio and microwave frequencies are causing significant damage to our cells, resulting in extreme increases in autism, heart irregularities, brain wave changes, cancer, and generational fertility destruction in males, but even more significantly in females.

The most prominent changes due to Wi-Fi radiation, though, are in our children and teenagers due to their developing immune systems and thinner skeletal structures. As stated by university researchers, government scientists, and international scientific advisors, "A minimum of 57.7% of schoolgirls exposed to low-level microwave radiation (Wi-Fi) are at risk of suffering stillbirth, fetal abnormalities or genetically damaged children, when they give birth. Any genetic damage may pass to successive generations" (Trower, 2013). And, laptop and notebook computers that have Wi-Fi connections can also cause harm to sperm DNA (Bioinitiative Report, 2014).

Federal and global regulations only deal with thermal heat exposure caused by laptops and such. They completely ignore the real dangers of low-frequency radiation. An example to compare the two is that you can microwave your food, yet the inside of the box stays cool because radiation only cooks the food at the cellular level as opposed to a regular oven that heats the whole box with conventional heating.

## WHAT IS AN EMF?

Electromagnetic fields (EMF) are present everywhere in our environment but are invisible to the human eye. Electric fields are produced by the local build-up of electric charges in the atmosphere associated with thunderstorms. The earth's magnetic field causes a compass needle to orient in a north-south direction and is used by birds and fish for navigation.

Electromagnetic radiation consists of an electrical field plus a magnetic field. The two fields oscillate perpendicular to one another as they travel through space. Amplitude is the height or breath of the wave.

So frequency represents the waves per specific time frame, usually seconds, from extremely low frequency radiation (ELF), which have longer wavelengths (longer wavelengths are measured in megahertz), up to short gamma rays, in which the wavelengths are extremely close together. Rays with shorter wavelengths can carry more information and more energy.

There are two factors to consider with regard to wireless technologies: the radiation between handset and base station and the information-carrying radio wave (ICRW). Microwave radiation carries the voice/data information by means of modulations.

Scientists are now observing that pulsed information transfer by microwaves triggers biological effects. Even the lowest pulsed frequency might not be safe. Wireless technologies pulse radiation in an organized fashion, and these pulses interfere with the various biochemical processes going on in the body (Kuhn, Lott, Kramer, & Kuster, 2012).

Just as electromagnetic interference from wireless technologies interferes with an airplane's or a hospital's equipment, it can interfere with our inner processes. We are electrochemical/electromagnetic creatures, as can be experienced when we hook up to an electroencephalogram (EEG, a test that measures and records the electrical activity of the brain) or an electrocardiogram (EKG or ECG, a test that checks for problems with the electrical activity of the heart).

Since Wi-Fi is everywhere and everyone has sold out to its use, it is difficult to mitigate the effects. One way is to wire your homes with Ethernet cables, switch your phones back to old land lines, or order wireless phones that broadcast less radiation.

## EMF Sensitivity and Biological Effects

The media has created frenzy over the safety of exposure to EMF. Komando, in a special *USA Today* report (2014), states that she assumes the worst and takes steps to stay safe. We hear folks requesting "safe schools" in lieu of "smart schools." The interest in EMF sensitivity is not new; it is just more pronounced. We have generated greater awareness, and the public demands action.

## Smart Use of Technology

The good news is that most of us don't have to give up our smartphones if we use them wisely.

iPad, iPhone, Android phones, tablets, and video games are all signs of the times, and they're things that you cannot live without! Or can you? As I've discussed, Wi-Fi and cellular technology may be the most devastating threat to health yet in the form of EMFs, and one that industry, government, and wireless consumers don't like to acknowledge. But the threat is something that everyone needs to be aware of. Cellular phones present similar challenges for you and your family.

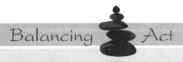

*Balancing Act*

## SO WHAT IS SMART USE?

- Text, don't talk, whenever possible.

- Use speaker mode to keep your phone as far away from your head as possible.

- Go offline. Turn off your cell phone when you're not using it and shut off your wireless router at night. (You'll be amazed how much more soundly you'll sleep.)

- Get your phone out of your pocket; men who carry their mobile there have lower sperm counts than those who don't carry a cell phone.

- Avoid tight spaces (buses, elevators, trains, and subways) where your phone has to work harder to get a signal through metal.

- Buy low, choosing a phone with a low SAR number.

- Replace your cordless phones with corded land line phones.

- Don't cradle your laptop; putting it on your lap exposes your reproductive organs to EMFs.

- Most important of all, restrict cell and cordless phone use during pregnancy. Heavy phone use during pregnancy has been linked to increased risk of miscarriage and birth defects. A 2008 survey of more than 13,000 children found that those whose mothers used a cell phone during pregnancy were more likely to have behavior problems, such as hyperactivity and trouble controlling their emotions.

- Don't rely on the many stick-on devices available for your cell phone or computer that claim to protect you.

But remember that even if you go back to wired technologies at home, Wi-Fi is expanding rapidly into schools and other public buildings. If the telecommunications industry has its way, we will all be bathed in a sea of artificial radiation from nonstop EMF exposure.

# Sick Building Syndrome

Amid the highest unemployment rate in recent decades and massive job losses around the country, most workers feel happy to at least be employed. What they aren't feeling, however, is healthy. One in three workers has at least one symptom of clinical depression; 41% say they feel stressed sometimes, often, or very often; and one in five has trouble falling asleep often or very often. In all, 14% are being treated for high cholesterol, and one in five is taking blood-pressure-lowering medication (APA, 2009).

Stress plays a key role, and, 75% to 90% of physician office visits are related to stress-induced symptoms (WebMD, 2012). *Why? How? What is going on?*

Headache, runny nose, itchy eyes, and more! Is this related to the cold and flu season, or are you well at home and sick at work? You may have what is known as Sick Building Syndrome. How do you know if you live or work in a "sick building"? The facts tell us that some of your symptoms might be due to the physical infrastructure, upholstery, or HVAC system of the building you work in. Other factors contributing to Sick Building Syndrome might include chemical fumes from things such as carpeting, office supplies like printers, computers, and desks. Depending on the type of work going on in the building, this risk could be higher for chemical problems. There also may be outdoor pollutants contributing from busy city streets or industrial parks, as well as biological contaminants in the building structure such as mold, mildew, dust mites, pollen, and viruses (Joshi, 2008).

Productivity is compromised, and safety is a challenge because our workforce is virtually unwell. We can do something about it, though. We can take a zero-tolerance approach! We can remove or modify pollutants, clean the air, increase ventilation rates, educate, and communicate!

Chronic neuroimmune disease is the term applied to dysfunction of both the immune and nervous systems. It is associated with symptoms such as chronic fatigue, nausea, vision problems, and memory loss (Tian, Ma, Kaarela, & Li, 2012). Both the World Health Organization (WHO) and the U.S. Environmental Protection Agency (EPA; Joshi, 2008) recognize Sick Building Syndrome and building-related illnesses as a public health challenge. We are exposed to hundreds of chemicals on a daily basis, and multiple-chemical sensitivity can be a problem.

# The Information Age at Work/Home/School

Regardless of our work environment, we are connected, sometimes far too often. We live in an information age, and it will continue to escalate. It has impacted the workforce by creating situations in which tasks are automated and sometimes by replacing physical workers with computers, robotics, and more. Think of it in terms of automation, productivity, and job loss. Even the information technology (IT) sector is not immune. Let's face it—industry is information-intensive.

Twitter, Facebook, eBooks, newsfeeds, and mobile apps are all sources of information that did not exist a few years ago, and they change the way in which we process information. We spend our time in "the cloud" where information is stored until we need it; the cloud has, in many cases, become our back-up system. Operating systems for our "devices" are updated, necessitating an increased number of more-efficient apps.

My backup is Dropbox, one of many applications that ensure peace of mind. I can see anything on my PC, my phone, or my iPad simply by going to Dropbox. It enables me to transfer very large files without a per-file fee; I can grant third-party access to my Dropbox account without having to share a password. And, those with whom I share find it very helpful.

There's an app that exists to do almost anything you might want. A must-have list might include the following:

| App | Benefits | Access |
|---|---|---|
| 1Password | Password management to store all logins and other private information | https://itunes.apple.com/us/app/1password-password-manager/id568903335?mt=8&ignmpt=uo%3D4 |
| Boxie | A filing system that works, thanks to bookmarks (shortcuts) to your most-used folders | https://itunes.apple.com/us/app/boxie-prettify-your-dropbox/id674521086?mt=8&ignmpt=uo%3D4 |
| Evernote | Stores notes, archived webpages, and pdf documents | https://itunes.apple.com/us/app/evernote/id281796108?mt=8&ignmpt=uo%3D4 |
| 30/30 | Your official To-Do list (but think of it as a Will-Do list!) | http://3030.binaryhammer.com/ |
| Mailbox | Puts email in its place to facilitate use and reminders | www.mailboxapp.com/ |

# You and Your Cellular Phone

Your cell phone is more than a constant companion; it knows everything about you. The National Security Agency (NSA) claims that collecting phone metadata does not tell the agency everything about you, but you and your calls may be tracked (Kaminski, 2014). You depend on your cellular technology; you even have a program that helps you to locate the phone if you misplace it.

What would you do without that phone? Could you function? There are many among us who are eliminating cell phone use due to health concerns and going back to the primitive landline. Whatever you decide to do, remember that there is an off switch to the device, and you do not need to be enslaved unless you choose to do so. You make the choice, and have the opportunity to create a life in balance.

# Social Media

Simply stated, social media "is interaction among people in which they create, share, or exchange information and ideas in virtual communities and networks" (www.google.com/#q=social+media+). It has become a science; it is big industry; and it continues to enhance our ability to communicate, but we need to know how much is too much.

## How Much Is Too Much?

How do you know when you have had enough? Are you overconnected to social media? Do you find the need to check your Facebook, Twitter, and LinkedIn accounts throughout the day? Can you divert your time and attention to activities that don't drain your balance? Can you use a program that posts for you once or twice weekly or twice daily in order to save time, energy, and exposure? What can you do to regain balance when it comes to social media and the choices that you make? See the "Aligning Yourself to Stay Connected and Safe" sidebar later in this chapter.

## How Does It Affect Career, Choices, and Compliance?

What can we do to tame our connectivity? How do we manage our time with the convenience of modern technology and respect for our health and our schedules? There are many things that can be done, but they all require commitment. It is like making a New Year's Resolution—should it be a resolution or a commitment?

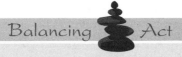

Balancing Act

## TAME YOUR ELECTRONIC MAIL

You can check your mail on your phone or tablet. Many people check their email even when they do not have time to handle everything in their inbox. Instead of this approach, try checking emails only during times you have set aside for handling them, never when you're rushing somewhere or have just a few minutes before a meeting. When you do check your email, read and handle the messages immediately. When looking at email, make one of the four following decisions:

1. Review the message once and act on it: delete it, file it, or forward it.

2. If a quick response is all that is needed, do it now and move on.

3. If needed, delegate the task to someone else.

4. If the email is project or task based, schedule a reminder via your email software to send an alert when the item is due.

Also take advantage of all the practical features of most email software packages. They may offer some form of electronic calendar, task lists, sticky notes, flags for follow-up and organizing, email reminders, and rules for automatically sorting and filing emails. For example, if you work with specific team members on a project, and the only emails you get from those team members relate to that project, you can tell your software to automatically send those messages to a folder that you will then manage during time set aside for that project. If your business or community education services offer courses on managing email software, take advantage of it to learn the best approaches to manage your technology tools.

Your goal should be to manage content without chaos. Don't allow the technology to rule your life. Instead, allow the technology to contribute to work/life balance by making your time yours alone.

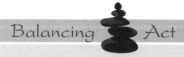
*Balancing Act*

# MASTERING YOUR OWN TECHNOLOGY

Are you master of technology such as email and cell phones, or is technology the master of you? Try this self-assessment to see where you fall.

Answer each question yes or no.

1. I organize myself before placing a telephone call.

2. I schedule telephone conversations to avoid playing phone tag.

3. If I have a complicated question, I call the person instead of sending an email.

4. If I am exchanging multiple emails on a single issue, I call instead of continuing to email.

5. I set time to respond to my email instead of interrupting my work for each one.

6. I keep my contacts list up to date with email, phone, and fax, so I can easily contact those I need to reach.

7. I use an electronic calendar to keep track of my appointments.

8. I use a contact relationship management (CRM) system like Constant Contact from InfusionSoft to manage my mail, contacts, and sequence messaging.

9. I update my voicemail and email so people can reach me before problems get out of hand, including using autoresponders indicating that I am out of the office.

10. I turn off my cell phone (or put it on vibrate if I'm expecting an important call) when at a restaurant.

11. I take the appropriate time to learn new technology systems or devices *before* trying to implement them.

The more you answer yes, the more you are in control of technology.

*Adapted from Womack, 2011.*

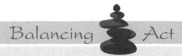

Balancing Act

# Aligning Yourself to Stay Connected and Safe

You can balance social media engagement and avoid becoming addicted. How you do that depends on your job, your community, your social circle, and your need for connectivity. Can social media be a part of your work performance? The answer is yes, if its use is work-related. In order to balance connectivity and safety, consider these principles:

1. Use social media to educate the communities you serve.

2. Have a plan for how often you connect and with whom.

3. Avoid becoming consumed with the need to post.

4. Tweets are done in real-time; feel free to retweet appropriately.

5. Be flexible and use time blocks that are self-imposed.

6. Don't be afraid to search the Internet to learn how to achieve a task. This is my personal secret to productivity and efficiency. After all, why try to reinvent the wheel when someone has already produced a YouTube video to show you how to do it?

7. Create an editorial calendar and stick with it to track your posts, time, and attention.

8. Increase your efficiency with tools and apps.

9. Remember that life goes on and do not limit your communications to online only.

10. Take a deep breath and relax; you would do that in verbal communication—so do it online as well.

# Downtime

Downtime—we are all too familiar with it. We think of downtime as a slow server, an app that is not responding, or a social network that is not up and running. Before the days of social media and connectivity, we took the time for personal downtime. And, guess what—we should still do so. We do not need to use the phone when walking from one location to another or crossing the street. There are so few sacred spaces that are untouched by the Internet and more.

Perhaps it is time for a "creative pause" or disengagement. Our need for belonging is cited in Maslow's hierarchy of needs. Think of how it would feel to stop belonging for a few minutes of your time, to forget your "followers" for 30 to 60 minutes, or to stop liking every post that you see merely because it is indicative of belonging. Downtime is a good thing!

# HEALTH IMPACT

Sites like Facebook, Twitter, and Instagram were created to connect users and enhance interaction; many research studies demonstrate that the opposite is true (Correa, 2010). Those who rely heavily on social media throughout the day can experience detachment, boredom, and perhaps loneliness. A constant need to connect with what is happening around the corner or across the globe can prevent one from remaining present in the environment. Think about the time that you spend on these sites and the positive or negative effect on your own health. Only you know how it affects your state of well-being.

# PERFORMANCE IMPACT

In 2012 Americans spent approximately 20% of their time on social medial while in the workplace (Federman, 2013). That number has certainly increased. Is there a possible link between constant use of social media and job or academic performance? How does texting affect productivity? Are all connections while at work job-related, or are you shopping online? Is your research work-related or it is personal? Can employees be trusted to use social media in the workplace? Look at the most visited, time-wasting sites:

- Social media: 14%
- Online shopping: 12%
- Entertainment/lifestyle: 8%
- Sports: 3%
- Travel: 2%

And, of those time-wasters, Facebook tops the list, followed by LinkedIn, Google+, Amazon, ESPN, YouTube, Twitter, Craigslist, and Pinterest.

Do we depend on the click of a mouse rather than human communication, and how does that affect relationships? Think about it—and be honest with yourself—has social media interfered with your own work performance?

Years ago I worked at a major medical school, and classrooms were set aside for medical students to watch their hospital-related soap operas during the day. I never quite understood the philosophy, and I often wondered if that is where the true "practice" of medicine was learned. Have we done the same thing with the internet and social media (Kaplan & Heinlein, 2010)?

In this chapter, we talked about putting technology in its place. You now know the impact of connectivity on your health and that of your family, and you know how to recognize the symptoms that could result in long-term effects. From EMFs to Sick Building Syndrome, you have discovered an awareness of technology that you did not have before. So, how much is too much, and what do you now need to do to find your balance?

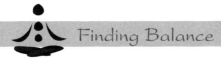 Finding Balance

## REFLECTIONS

- Use connectivity efficiently to increase productivity, avoid downtime, and maximize performance.

- Use connectively wisely to avoid overexposure to possible harmful effects.

- Know your body and monitor your response.

- Remember the off switch and use it as needed.

- Be aware of the challenges of connectivity.

# References

Aldad, T. S., Gan, G., Gao, X., & Taylor, H. S. (2012). Fetal radiofrequency radiation exposure from 800-1900 Mhz-rated cellular telephones affects neurodevelopment and behavior in mice. *Scientific Reports 2*, article number 312. Retrieved from http://www.nature.com/srep/2012/120315/srep00312/full/srep00312.html

American Psychological Association (APA). (2009). Stress in America 2009. Retrieved from https://www.apa.org/news/press/releases/stress/2009/stress-exec-summary.pdf

Apple. (2014). 1984-Macintosh. The computer that changed everything. Retrieved from www.apple.com/30-years/1984/

Bioinitiative Report. (23 March 2014). EMF risks - Wifi dangers - protection - news and information. Retrieved from http://www.emf-risks.com/

Centers for Disease Control and Prevention (CDC). (2013). Frequently asked questions about cell phones and your health. Retrieved from http://www.cdc.gov/nceh/radiation/factsheets/224613_FAQ_Cell%20Phones%20and%20Your%20Health.pdf

Copes, R. (2011). Wireless technology: A risk to health. *British Columbia Medical Journal, 53*(4), 198-199.

Correa, T., Hinsley, A. W., & De Zuniga, H. G. (2010). Who interacts on the Web?: The intersection of users' personality and social media use. *Computers in Human Behavior, 26*(2), 247-253.

Dean, A. L., Rea, W. J., Smith, C. W., & Barrier, A. L. (n.d.). Electromagnetic and radiofrequency fields effect on human health. American Academy of Environmental Medicine. Retrieved at http://aaemonline.org/emf_rf_position.html

Fathi, E., & Farahzadi, R. (2014). Interaction of mobile telephone radiation with biological systems in veterinary and medicine. *Journal of Biomedical Engineering and Technology, 2*(1), 1-4. Retrieved from http://pubs.sciepub.com/jbet/2/1/1/jbet-2-1-1.pdf

Federman, E. (2013). Internet social networks increase workplace productivity. *Social Media Today.* Retrieved from http://socialmediatoday.com/elifed/1191686/internal-social-networks-increase-workplace-productivity

Funk, R. H. W., Monsees, T., & Ozkucur, N. (2009). Electromagnetic fields—from cell biology to medicine. *Science Direct: Progress in Histochemistry and Cytochemistry 43*, 177-264. Retrieved from http://www.google.com/url?sa=t&rct=j&q=&esrc=s&frm=1&source=web&cd=5&ved=0CD8QFjAE&url=http%3A%2F%2Fwww.researchgate.net%2Fpublication%2F23938298_Electromagnetic_effects_-_From_cell_biology_to_medicine%2Ffile%2F9c9605253fcdcb1c7b.pdf&ei=II-bU-TFDKSk8QHHjIDQDA&usg=AFQjCNENg3_DeXgwPHT7V5O2TCOlJmY91Q

Joshi, S. M. (2008). The sick building syndrome. *Indian Journal of Occupational and Environmental Medicine*, 12(2), 61-64. Retrieved from http://www.ncbi.nlm. nih.gov/pmc/articles/PMC2796751/

Kaminski, M. (2014, March 18). NSA surveillance program reaches 'into the past' to retrieve, replay phone calls. *The Washington Post*. Retrieved from www. washingtonpost.com/world/national-security/nsa-surveillance-program-reaches-into-the-past-to-retrieve-replay-phone-calls/2014/03/18/226d2646-ade9-11e3-a49e-76adc9210f19_story.html

Kaplan, A. M., & Heinlein, M. (2010). Users of the world, unite! Challenges and opportunities of social media. *Business Horizons, 53*(1), 59-68.

Komando, K. (2014, May 30). Do cellphones cause radiation? *USA Today.* Retrieved from http://www.usatoday.com/story/tech/columnist/komando/2014/05/30/cellphone-radiation/9566879/

Kuhn, S., Lott, U., Kramer, A., & Kuster, N. (2012). Assessment of human exposure to electromagnetic radiation from wireless devices in home and office environments. Retrieved from www.who.int/peh-emf/meetings/archive/bsw_kuster.pdf

Miller, B. H. (2011). The death of secrecy: need to know...with whom to share. Center for the Study of Intelligence. CSI Publications, 3(55). Retrieved from https://www.cia.gov/library/center-for-the-study-of-intelligence/csi-publications/csi-studies/studies/vol.-55-no.-3/the-death-of-secrecy-need-to-know...with-whom-to-share.html

Tian, L., Ma, L., Kaarela, T., & Li, Z. (2012). Neuroimmune crosstalk in the central nervous system and its significance for neurological diseases. *Journal of Neuroinflammation, 9*(1), 155.

Trower, B. (24 August, 2013). WiFi report: Humanity at the brink. Retrieved from http://rense.com/general96/trower.html U.S. Food and Drug Administration. (2012). Health issues: Do cell phones post a health hazard? Retrieved from http://www.fda.gov/Radiation-EmittingProducts/RadiationEmittingProductsandProcedures/HomeBusinessandEntertainment/CellPhones/ucm116282.htm

U.S. Food and Drug Administration (2012). Health Issues: do cell phones post a health hazard? Retrieved from http://www.fda.gov/Radiation-EmittingProducts/RadiationEmittingProductsandProcedures/HomeBusinessandEntertainment/CellPhones/ucm116282.htm

Volkow, N. D., Tomasi, D., Wang, G-J., Vaska, P., Fowler, J. S., Telang, F.,...Wong, C. (2011). Effects of cell phone radiofrequency signal exposure on brain glucose metabolism. *Journal of the American Medical Association, 305*(8), 808.

WebMD. (2012). The effects of stress on your body. Retrieved from http://www.webmd.com/mental-health/effects-of-stress-on-your-body

Womack, J. (2011). Three tips for saving time on email. *Entrepreneur.* Retrieved from http://www.entrepreneur.com/article/220424

# PART II
## FINDING AND KEEPING BALANCE

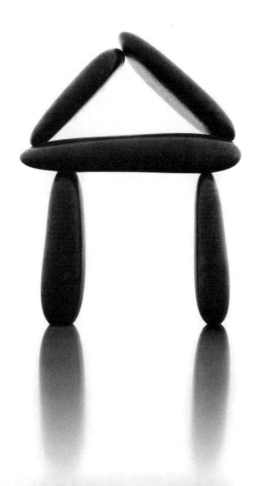

*"The body says what words cannot."*

*—Martha Graham*

# 7

# FATIGUE

*—Sharon M. Weinstein, MS, RN, CRNI, FACW, FAAN*

Clear thinking, critical thinking, and clear communication are imperatives in all employees and in all professions. We are challenged more than ever before with the effect of fatigue on outcomes. Fatigue is a reality in nursing. Every day, during every shift, nurses can experience fatigue of their minds, bodies, and spirits. Workload, work hours, work structures, and many other factors can indirectly or directly cause fatigue in multiple industries and affect safety. Regardless of the profession, fatigue takes its toll and has affected physicians, nurses, police, firefighters, emergency personnel, fighter pilots, naval crews, and transportation workers—all of whom work in environments where the timing of work is not always conveniently matched to the human circadian rhythm, and the length of the work may challenge one's ability to function safely (Dorrian, Lamond, & Dawson, 2000).

Within the healthcare setting one of today's greatest challenges is delivering safer care in complex, fast-moving environments. We recognize that in such environments things often can, and do, go wrong. Adverse events occur, and unintentional but serious harm comes to patients during routine clinical practice or as a result of a clinical decision.

# Fatigue Defined

Fatigue is mental or physical exhaustion that stops a person from being able to function normally. However, fatigue is more than just feeling tired or drowsy. You may often become tired through physical or mental effort; that is not unusual. When you are so weary that you cannot go on, that is true fatigue.

Fatigue is a factor that has been linked to stress, safety, and performance decrements in numerous work environments (Leung, Chan, Ng, & Wong, 2006).

Fatigue can be physical or psychological—or a combination of the two—and can lead to compromised decision-making, reaction time, and critical thinking; it can also negatively influence general health (Drake, Luna, George, & Steege, 2012). Within the healthcare sector, where the commodity with which we deal is human lives and human happiness, there is great concern about fatigue. In December 2011, The Joint Commission (TJC) issued a Sentinel Event Alert, "Health Care Worker Fatigue and Patient Safety," which identified that shift length and work schedules were found to have a significant impact on healthcare workers' quantity and quality of sleep (TJC, 2011).

## How Does It Feel?

The effects of fatigue increase with age. Those older than 50 years of age tend to have lighter, fragmented sleep, which can prevent them from receiving the recuperative effects from a full night of sleep and can make them more likely to become fatigued. Lack of sleep has been indirectly linked with mental and physical disorders, as well as what we refer to as "total fatigue."

### Mental Fatigue

Anxiety and depression can be triggered or made worse by fatigue and irregular sleep patterns. Neurobehavioral effects include behavioral lapses (error of omission), false responses (error of commission), learning, and recall deficits. Mental fatigue levels may be influenced by mental and emotional demands in the workplace. The Mayo Clinic staff (2014) identifies psychological conditions such as anxiety, depression, grief, and stress as factors in mental fatigue.

## Physical Fatigue

We may be physically drained, and we do not know why. Could it be the work schedule or the work setting in which we operate? Could it be due to the challenges we face at home and perhaps the fact that each of our days has more than 24 hours? According to Barker and Nussbaum (2011), fatigue-induced sleep and rest habits may contribute to:

- Coronary heart disease (blocked arteries in the heart)
- Ischemic heart disease (blocked arteries leading to lack of oxygen to the heart muscle)
- High blood pressure
- Myocardial infarction (heart attack)

Our sensitive digestive tracts are designed to consume and absorb food at regular intervals. Shiftwork, not taking time for meals, and lack of hydration are known to contribute to:

- Bowel habit changes
- Digestive complaints
- Increased risk of peptic (stomach) ulcers

Fatigue and irregular sleep patterns have been associated with a number of negative effects for pregnant women and fertility rates, including:

- Increased risk of miscarriage
- Low birth-weight babies
- A higher occurrence of premature births

## Adrenal Fatigue

Adrenal fatigue is a collection of signs and symptoms, often known as a "syndrome" that occurs when the adrenal glands function below the necessary level. The greatest contributor to this common health challenge is stress, and stress is often associated with fatigue! "Fatigue" is a part of the label, and although you might not exhibit obvious signs of an illness, you live and function while feeling unwell. Does your day begin with coffee or carbonated beverages/energy drinks because you need a lift of some kind?

Adrenal fatigue has had many names, including non-Addison's hypo-adrenia, adrenal neurasthenia, and adrenal apathy. Although conventional (Western) medicine does not recognize it, millions of people are affected by it. Remember that the world of healthcare relies on "coding," and if there is no code associated with a syndrome, it is not billable; thus, it does not exist. Try telling that to those who face this challenge each and every day.

Adrenal fatigue can wreak havoc with your life. In more serious cases, the activity of the adrenal glands is so diminished that you may have dif-ficulty getting out of bed for more than a few hours per day. Other organs and systems can become affected. Changes occur in your carbohydrate, protein, and fat metabolism; fluid and electrolyte balance; heart and car-diovascular system; and even libido. Although your body does its best to compensate, it does not always succeed. The adrenal glands retaliate by mobilizing your body's stress responders through hormones that regulate energy production and storage, immune function, heart rate, muscle tone, and other processes that enable you to cope with the stress (Mayo Clinic Staff, 2014). The result is that you are wiped out!

## Total Fatigue

Those who are fatigued exhibit lack of energy, apathy, inattention, diffi-culty concentrating, poor decision-making, lack of initiative, indifference, irritability, ptosis (eye irritation), slow reaction time, and poor commu-nication. Physiologic effects of fatigue include insulin resistance, poor arousal response, and hypoxemia. Total fatigue refers to a state comprised of both dimensions: mental and physical. Over time, this may contribute to an inability to function at normal capacity and can lead to an increased risk of injury or error (WebMD, 2013).

"How many inner resources one needs to tolerate a life of leisure without fatigue."

–Natalie Clifford Barney

# Who Owns Fatigue?

Registered nurses and employers share the responsibility of implementing strategies to reduce risks from shiftwork and long work hours. Stakeholders who have a contractual relationship with the worksite and influence work hours also have a responsibility to promote safe and healthy work hours. An optimal work environment proactively addresses fatigue and promotes wellness. The American Nurses Association (ANA, 2014a) supports the health and well-being of the nurse and promotes strategies to reduce the risks of working while fatigued.

## Employer Responsibility

The employer can do much to shift the paradigm and create a culture of safety, wellness, and caring. Clear and compelling visions start us along a path of generating a future we deserve to have. In the healthcare setting, everyone assumes responsibility for patient safety and good outcomes. Nurses might argue that they own safety, but it is clear that certain factors can and do contribute to fatigue on the part of employers/management (Hendren, 2011; Lerman et al., 2012; Reed, 2013). Even the best designed fatigue-management plans cannot regulate sleep behaviors during one's rest periods and days off.

Any approach to addressing workplace fatigue must include collaboration among management and staff. In the healthcare setting, an assessment of current staffing, scheduling, and acuity levels is needed to avoid unsafe circumstances. Self-scheduling is perceived as an advantage on the part of nurses; however, the nurse who chooses to work 72 hours in a workweek is following the path to fatigue. Autonomy might win, but the human body fails. Recommendations for identifying and addressing fatigue-related risks include the following:

- Assess your fatigue-related risks—staffing, consecutive shifts, off-shift hours.

- Develop a plan to include education, strategies, and role modeling.

- Invite staff input in designing work schedules.

- Create and implement an alertness management plan.

- Provide nonpunitive opportunities for staff to express concerns about fatigue.

- Encourage teamwork to support staff who work long hours.

- Develop an internal system to monitor and report fatigue levels.

Promoting a positive, safe, work environment reduces the risk for job stress and the associated difficulties with not getting enough sleep. Safe levels of staffing are essential to providing a safer environment for all workers, especially those with responsibility for patient care. With fair compensation, staff will be less compelled to seek supplemental income through overtime, extra shifts, and other practices that are known to contribute to worker fatigue.

## CONTRIBUTING FACTORS TO WORKPLACE FATIGUE

Lack of organizational support

Changes in leadership

The frequency of change itself

Decision dilemma

The 24/7/360 nature of the business

Inability to find/retain top talent

Daily change in priorities

Fewer resources combined with greater expectations

Exhaustion

Lack of a healing environment

Putting out fires

## EMPLOYEE RESPONSIBILITY

Any employee is responsible for practicing healthy behaviors that reduce the risk for working while fatigued or sleepy, result in arriving to work alert and well rested, and promote a safe commute to and from work. This is true regardless of the industry in which one works! This responsibility might require that you reject a work assignment that compromises the availability of sufficient time for sleep and recovery from work—for example, when your shift ends at midnight, and you are expected to return to work, fully rested, by 7:00 a.m. We all have different recovery times. Our bodies and minds are unique, and this concept often involves scheduled shifts and mandatory or voluntary overtime. It is everyone's responsibility to address one's own, as well as coworker, fatigue. Employees must be responsible and know their limits.

## WORK-RELATED AND NON-WORK-RELATED CONTRIBUTORS TO PERFORMANCE IMPAIRMENT

| Work-Related | Non-Work-Related |
| --- | --- |
| Work schedule | Quantity of sleep |
| Actual hours worked, including overtime and additional shifts | Quality of sleep |
| Type of work involved | Absence or presence of sleep disorders |
| Work environment | Existing health issues |

"I'm a workaholic, so I ignore the signs of fatigue and just keep going and going, and then conk out when I get home. It can be pretty stressful."

–Keke Palmer

## System Responsibility

The outcome is only as good as the system. And the system has been created to ensure positive outcomes.

---

## Ten Tips for Ensuring Organizational Leadership and Commitment to the System

---

Attach a sense of urgency

Partner with staff to ensure consistency of policy and procedures

Create a collaborative work environment

Educate and empower staff

Identify the areas and practices that may result in staff fatigue

Prioritize fatigue countermeasures and monitor effectiveness

Evaluate staffing and scheduling practices

Offer opportunity for feedback and ideas for improvement

Engage staff in recruitment and retention activities and
promote innovative strategies

Follow the system

---

What should a leader do? The leader should find and fix problems, make safety a core value, partner with others to make minimizing fatigue a priority, and measure the results, making adjustments as needed.

# Fatigue and Performance

We want to do the best job possible. We want to perform at the highest level. We want to succeed. Sometimes the environment itself impairs our ability to do so. When I worked in Eastern Europe, my nurse colleagues did not have healthy work environments. At the time, they worked without electricity, without an emergency generator, without adequate food for patients and staff, and in less-than-desirable conditions. I still recall seeing a full-term infant pass away because it wasn't possible to control the baby's body temperature in a nursery that was as cold inside as it was outside. But the nurses, with conviction, did what needed to be done; they performed at their best.

## BEST PRACTICES

In the words of a Thomas the Train song, "Accidents happen," but they should not be routine! Fatigue contributes to errors, but errors can be avoided by initiating and adhering to best practices.

Best practices are aimed at creating a system-wide approach to safety and the creation of a safe environment that supports open dialogue about errors, their causes, and strategies for prevention. Analysis of errors is a best practice, and corrective action naturally follows.

## PROVIDING A WELLNESS ENVIRONMENT

There is no doubt that a healthy, healing work environment is conducive to staff satisfaction, optimum performance, and good results. By embracing a workplace of wellness—replete with circles of wellness in which staff may relax, rejuvenate, and rejoice—we take the first step toward total wellness. Staff feels appreciated, valued, and recognized in a meaningful way.

It has increasingly become the responsibility of employers to provide preventative wellness programs to counter increasing costs and loss of productivity in the interest of the organization's bottom line. Such benefits not only increase the motivation and physical well-being of existing employees, but those benefits also become a differentiating factor to attract qualified new employees.

To create a workplace of wellness you need to:

- Capture senior-level support.
- Create a Wellness Committee or Council.
- Collect baseline information so that you can create a plan.

- Develop a yearly operating plan that is strategically linked to the institution's overall plan.

- Choose appropriate health initiatives consistent with your risk appraisals and claims history.

- Develop a supportive atmosphere.

- Model healthy behaviors by walking the walk and talking the talk.

- Monitor your outcomes and effect on the organization.

## Transparent Communication and Impact on Safety

Communication is at the very core of safety. Effective communication between management and staff is essential to keep everyone informed and involved in the culture of safety. Regardless of the goal, all internal communications should follow a strategic plan to be successful. Employees are more likely to be engaged in the results if they feel involved. In nursing, staff members seek a leader with a transformational style. Staff members prefer not to be micromanaged; they want to be embraced for the value that they bring to the clinical setting, engaged actively, and empowered to succeed. Today's transformational leaders have shifted from "management" to "leadership." They are able to identify the changes needed, guide the change by inspiring followers, and create a sense of commitment to change. What better way is there to promote a positive, professional work environment? After all, if our end goal is to find and keep balance, we need to first find ourselves in a positive, professional work setting. We need to be led, not managed, and transparent communication allows that to happen.

## Reduced Performance

High levels of fatigue cause reduced performance and productivity and increase the risk of accidents and injuries. Fatigue affects the ability to think clearly. As a result, people who are fatigued are unable to gauge their own level of impairment. They are unaware that they are not functioning as well or as safely as they would be if they were not fatigued. A number of real-world mishaps have resulted from performance failures associated with operator sleepiness (Caldwell, Caldwell, & Schmidt, 2008). This is certainly true of the transportation industry.

Performance levels drop as work periods become longer and sleep loss increases. Staying awake for 17 hours has the same effect on performance as having a blood alcohol content of 0.05%. Staying awake for 21 hours is equivalent to a blood alcohol content of 0.1% (Lamond & Dawson, 1999). The most common effects associated with fatigue are:

- Sleepiness
- Lack of concentration
- Impaired recall
- Irritability
- Poor judgment
- Reduced ability to communicate with others
- Reduced fine motor skills and hand-eye coordination
- Reduced visual perception
- Slower response times

Rogers (2012) studied the impact of fatigue on officers of the law. Not only do these effects decrease performance and productivity within the workplace, but they simultaneously increase the potential for incidents and injuries to occur. Fatigued workers may place themselves and others at risk in the following situations:

- When operating machinery (including driving vehicles)
- When performing critical tasks that require a high level of concentration
- Where the consequence of error is serious, including death or disaster

In the past, the 40-hour workweek was routine. Law enforcement agencies typically deployed their patrol officers based on that schedule, followed by 2 days off. More recently, some agencies have adopted a compressed workweek (CWW) schedule in which officers work four 10-hour shifts per week or three 12-hour shifts plus adjusted time to equal 40 hours (Bambra, Whitehead, Sowden, Akers, & Petticrew, 2008). This certainly is not new to the health professions.

Even the National Transportation Safety Board (NTSB) has analyzed fatigue-related factors in accidents on domestic air carriers. And the media has focused on truck-driver fatigue-related accidents. Is the fatigued officer, pilot, driver, or healthcare provider fit for duty?

Standards and regulations to promote patient safety and resident alertness have addressed the number of hours worked. While resident working hours have been a topic of discussion for years, nurse fatigue and hours worked have also been studied extensively. The ANA Nurse Fatigue Panel, of which I am a part, has developed a position paper on fatigue (ANA, 2014b). However, by focusing on the hour factor alone, we neglect what we know about sleep and performance that could influence multiple human factors. The Institute of Medicine (IOM, 2008) report on resident duty hours included a recommendation for 5-hour naps. As a student nurse, I recall many interns and residents napping on a stretcher in the hallway of our hospital wards; they did what they could to recover from fatigue.

Are mistakes caused by people or machinery? Think about how many times you have sought online support for a computer transaction—perhaps for an insurance claim. The "live" voice at the end of the line indicated that the "computer" made the mistake; we know all too well that the human being at the keyboard was the culprit.

A study found that four out of eight officers involved in on-the-job accidents and injuries were impaired because of fatigue (Dorrian et al., 2011). Such accidents include automobile crashes that were due to officers' impaired eye-hand coordination and a tendency to nod off behind the wheel. Other work-related injuries come from accidents that occur when officers have impaired balance and coordination.

## Drowsy Driving

We have all experienced dozing off in a classroom—perhaps because of a boring instructor. We may also have experienced dozing off while driving a car because it was too warm or because we were exhausted. I know many folks who have been in accidents in which they hit the car in front of them simply because of tiredness. They may have opened the windows to allow cool air to enter the vehicle or cranked up the music to stay awake and hopefully to make it home safely. Singing, talking on the phone, slapping yourself in the face, and keeping a full bladder are all tactics that tired workers have used to keep themselves awake while driving home. Never say to yourself, "I am almost there; I can make it home." It is no secret that one cannot and should not drive or operate machinery while tired.

## CHARACTERISTICS OF DROWSY-DRIVING CRASHES

Most drowsy-driving crashes happen between midnight and 6:00 a.m., when the body's need for sleep is greatest, and in the mid-afternoon (during the circadian dip).

The driver, who is probably male, is alone.

Sleep-related crashes tend to involve a single vehicle running off a high-speed road to the right or to the left.

Many drowsy-driving crashes involve serious injuries and/or fatalities.

The driver is often sleep deprived or fatigued.

Long distances without breaks are involved.

The trip includes driving through the night or mid-afternoon.

The driver has worked more than 60 hours per week or perhaps works multiple jobs.

A small amount of alcohol may contribute to the problem.

The driver may be taking over-the-counter or prescription cold tablets, antihistamines, or antidepressants.

*Adapted from http://www.nhtsa.gov/Impaired*

Tragically, drowsy driving has taken far too many lives. Traffic crashes are the leading cause of death of young people in the United States, taking the lives of at least 5,600 teens each year according to the National Highway Traffic Safety Administration (NHTSA, 2013). And, each year drowsy-driving crashes result in at least 1,550 deaths, 71,000 injuries, and $12.5 billion in monetary losses. Unfortunately, many people do not realize how tired they are, and they do not think about the fact that their skills are reduced when they are sleep-deprived. If you are a truck driver or shift worker planning to catch up on some sleep this weekend, it might be wise to rethink exactly how you're going to do that. Sleep must be a priority, like diet, water, and exercise.

# COMPASSION FATIGUE

Compassion fatigue is a combination of physical, emotional, and spiritual exhaustion associated with the care of patients with significant pain and physical distress (Lombardo & Eyre, 2011).

## SYMPTOMS OF COMPASSION FATIGUE

| Work-Induced | Physical | Emotional |
|---|---|---|
| Fear of working with specific clients/patients | Headaches | Mood swings and lack of focus |
| Decreased ability to feel empathy toward patient/family | Digestive problems | Restlessness or irritability |
| More frequent use of available sick days | Sleep challenges | Extreme sensitivity |
| Lack of joy | Fatigue | Anxiety and memory issues |

| Lack of defined purpose (see Chapter 1) | Muscle tension or aches | Substance abuse |
| --- | --- | --- |
| | Cardiac symptoms, palpitations | Depression, anger |

## Identifying Compassion Fatigue

In any setting in which care is provided, compassion fatigue is a possibility. Mental health professionals, preceptors, and others can help to validate the presence of compassion fatigue. Awareness of the problem is critical to developing an intervention. As a student, I recall attempting to be all things to all people. We had no label for it at the time, but I was a candidate for compassion fatigue. I did not take a day off because I wanted to be there to feed a patient who was dependent on me. I took home patients' laundry, and I did everything above and beyond the call of duty to provide care and service.

Triggers for compassion fatigue include:

- Evaluation of the work setting and conditions
- A tendency to become over involved
- Usual coping strategies and management of life crises
- Methods of self-care, if any, including massage, meditation, deep breathing
- Interest in enhancing personal and professional well-being

## Interventions

Now that you are aware of the issue of compassion fatigue, either for yourself or a staff member, it is so important to intervene in some way. Simply talking about one's feelings can be the first step. Be cognizant of resources within the work setting. Most employers have an Employee Assistance Program (EAP) as a part of the talent management or human resources department. EAPs can offer supportive counseling for either personal or work-related concerns. The EAP may provide lifestyle courses that address life-learning topics, such as managing time, balancing a budget, caring for an aging parent, communicating effectively, and reducing stress. These classes are designed to decrease stress, enhance work-life balance, and provide help for employees experiencing conditions such as compassion fatigue. See Chapter 8 for more on EAPs.

## DEALING WITH COMPASSION FATIGUE

How do we deal with the challenges? Some examples of helpful strategies might include changing work assignments or shifts; recommending time off or reducing overtime hours; encouraging attendance at a conference or personal development program; or becoming involved in a project of interest. These actions could contribute to work satisfaction, work balance, and a healthy attitude.

## EMBRACING FATIGUE

We all need downtime. We all need positive self-care strategies and healthy rituals to cope with something like compassion fatigue. This includes activities that replenish personal energy levels and enhance overall well-being. A commitment to taking care of oneself includes having adequate nutrition, hydration, sleep, and exercise. The nurse may need to be encouraged to try a new approach to self-care, such as a yoga class, massage, meditation, or Tai-Chi. Some facilities have onsite relaxation or respite centers where staff may unwind. They may offer Reiki, light massage, or a healing touch treatment. If an entire area cannot be designated, perhaps a room can be transformed by adding soothing colors to the walls and providing calming music, a waterfall, and comfortable seating.

## ALARM FATIGUE

Imagine the number of bells and whistles that are going off during a single shift. Hospitals are replete with noise; it is certainly not the place to go for an extended rest! Medical device alarms contribute to an environment that poses a significant risk to patient safety and anticipated outcomes.

Alarm fatigue is a national problem, specifically within the healthcare arena. The challenge with alarm desensitization is complex and relates to high false alarm rates, lack of standardization, and the plethora of alarming devices in clinical settings today.

## Outcomes and Impact

What are the hazards and how do they affect outcomes? Medical devices generate enough false alarms to create a reduction in response known as the "cry wolf effect." Frequent alarms are distracting and interfere with thought processes; they may even lead to staff disabling important alarm systems. We know that we do not want to miss a beat; alarms are designed for high sensitivity so that this is possible. When the alarm is viewed as a nuisance, it may be ignored. What was intended to make the healthcare environment safer has now generated the opposite effect. Organizations committed to finding solutions have formed interdisciplinary alarm management teams to assess the risk and identify safe strategies for alarm reduction.

# Injury

In addition to increased risk for errors and reduced job performance, drowsy driving and fatigue have major implications on the health of workers, especially nurses. Substantial scientific evidence links shift work and long hours to sleep disturbances, injuries, gastrointestinal and mood disorders, obesity, metabolic syndrome, cardiovascular disease, cancer, and adverse reproductive outcomes (Antunes, Levandovski, Dantas, Caumo, & Hidalgo, 2010; Brown et al., 2010; Bushnell, Colombi, Caruso, & Tak, 2010), some of which I discuss in more detail in the next few sections.

Fatigued workers need rest, breaks (including biological breaks), and time away from the workplace. The need for sleep is the second most powerful urge of the human body; it's second only to the need to breathe. Imagine how you might feel and function after 24 sleepless hours. People aren't designed for 24/7 operations. Work-related injuries are not a required part of the job; we all need balance between activity and recovery time in order to prevent injury. Repetitive work without regular breaks or rest can contribute to strains, sprains, poor posture, headaches, stress, and, of course, fatigue. Injuries may possibly be reduced by enforcing:

- Regular breaks and scheduled meal times
- Regular working hours
- Regular time away from the job, even if just for a few minutes (perhaps for a walk around the grounds)

# GASTROINTESTINAL AND MOOD DISORDERS

When we are exhausted, we are often too tired to eat. Our mood changes and we are irritable. This is fatigue at its worst. There is a direct link between blood sugar and mood. Carbohydrates are broken down into glucose and your brain runs on this type of fuel. The more unsteady your blood sugar supply, the more uneven your mood. Avoid overconsumption of "bad mood foods" such as wheat, rye, and barley. Gluten sensitivity may contribute to diarrhea, constipation, bloating, and other digestive challenges, even in the absence of diagnosed Celiac disease (Strawbridge, 2013).

The good news is that just as eating the wrong things (or not eating) can negatively effect your energy level and mood, taking in enough of the right things can help you. Let's face it—what you eat will impact your ability to be well and to stay well; it will impact balance. You may have heard, "Give the body the right tools and it will do its best work." It is true because making smart choices can boost both your mental and physical health.

There is good news, and that is that we do not have to think of achieving good health with drugs alone. There are natural solutions that I have used for years, and there are studies within the literature that attest to the benefits of a more holistic approach to well-being (Ernst, 2007; National Prevention Council, 2011). Let's examine some of those approaches and how they impact our health outcomes.

# BATTLING DEPRESSION WITHOUT DRUGS

Depression is a good starting point; when you view the drug advertisements in the media related to depression, you realize the depth of the health challenge. You also realize the depth of the toxicities and understand why the public seeks alternatives or more natural methods of coping. There have been six double-blind placebo controlled trials to date, five of which show merit. The first trial by Dr. Andrew Stoll from Harvard Medical School, published in the *Archives of General Psychiatry*, gave 40 depressed patients either omega-3 supplements or a placebo and found a highly significant improvement (Stoll et al., 1999). The next, published in *The American Journal of Psychiatry*, tested the effects of giving 20 people suffering from severe depression who were already on antidepressants but still depressed a highly concentrated form of omega-3 fat called ethyl-EPA versus a placebo. By the third week the depressed patients on the ethyl-EPA were showing major improvement in their moods whereas those on placebo were not (Nemets, Stahl, & Belmaker, 2002). A recent pooling of trials (a meta-analysis) which looked at all good quality trials of omega-3 fats and mood disorders concluded that omega-3 fats reduced depressive symptoms by an average of 53% and that there was as correlation between dose and depressive symptom improvement, meaning that higher dose omega-3 was more effective than a lower dose. Of those that measured the Hamilton Rating Scale, including one open trial that didn't involve placebos, the average improvement in depression was approximately double that shown by antidepressant drugs and without the side-effects (Khan, Khan, Shankles, & Polissar, 2002). This may be because omega-3 fats help to build the brain's neuronal (brain cell) connections as well as the receptor sites for neurotransmitters; therefore, the more omega-3 fats in your blood, the more serotonin you are likely to make and the more responsive you become to its effects (Agrawal & Gomez-Pinilla, 2012).

In terms of side effects, very occasionally, when starting omega-3 fish oil supplementation, some people can get slightly loose bowels or fish-tasting burps, but this is quite rare. Supplementing fish oils also reduces risk for heart disease, reduces arthritic pain, and may improve memory and concentration.

Both tryptophan and 5-HTP, both naturally occurring amino acids, have been shown to have an antidepressant effect in clinical trials, although 5-HTP is more effective (Turner, Loftis, & Blackwell, 2005). So how do tryptophan and 5-HTP compare with antidepressants? The natural approach may be better, simply because of decreased potential for side effects associated with drugs.

Because antidepressant drugs, in some sensitive people, can induce an overload of serotonin—a result called serotonin syndrome, which is characterized by feeling hot, having high blood pressure, and experiencing twitching and cramping of muscles, dizziness, and disorientation—a licensed independent practitioner should always direct the approach to care and monitor progress.

As for side effects, some people experience mild gastrointestinal disturbance on 5-HTP, which usually stops within a few days. Because there are serotonin receptors in the gut that don't normally expect to get the real thing so easily, they can overreact if the amount is too high, resulting in transient nausea. If so, it helps to lower the dose or take it with food.

Exercise, sunlight, and reducing your stress level also tend to promote serotonin production.

## AVOIDING SUGARS AND CARBOHYDRATES

Eating lots of sugar is going to give you sudden peaks and troughs in the amount of glucose in your blood, which can lead to symptoms that include fatigue, irritability, dizziness, insomnia, excessive sweating (especially at night), poor concentration and forgetfulness, excessive thirst, depression and crying spells, digestive disturbances, and blurred vision. Because the brain depends on an even supply of glucose, it is no surprise to find that sugar has been implicated in aggressive behavior, anxiety, depression, and fatigue.

Lots of refined sugar and refined carbohydrates (meaning white bread, pasta, rice, and most processed foods) is also linked with depression because these foods not only supply very little in the way of nutrients but they also use up the mood-enhancing B vitamins. (Turning each teaspoon of sugar into energy requires B vitamins.) In fact, a study of 3,456 middle-aged civil servants, published in *The British Journal of Psychiatry*, found that those who had a diet that contained a lot of processed foods had a 58% increased risk for depression, whereas those whose diet could be described as containing more whole foods had a 26% reduced risk for depression (Borchard, 2011).

The best way to keep your blood sugar level even is to eat what is called a low glycemic load (GL) diet and avoid, as much as you can, refined sugar and refined foods. Instead, eat whole foods, fruits, vegetables, and regular meals. The book, *The Low-GL Diet Bible* by Patrick Holford (2009) explains exactly how to do this, so that book is a great resource if you really want to improve your blood sugar balance. Caffeine also has a direct effect on your blood sugar and your mood and is best kept to a minimum, as is alcohol (Smith, Sutherland, & Christopher, 2005).

The best part of balancing your blood sugar—no side effects.

## Addressing Vitamin D Deficiencies

You are most at risk for vitamin D deficiency if you are elderly (because your ability to make it in the skin reduces with age), dark-skinned (you require up to six times more sunshine than a light-skinned person to make the same amount of vitamin D), overweight (your vitamin D stores may be tucked away within your fat tissue), or you tend to shy away from the sun by covering up and using sunblock. Of course, you should never risk your skin health by getting sunburned. The National Institute of Health Fact Sheets on Vitamin D offer quick facts and suggestions on handling deficiencies (2014). For example, vitamin D is readily available in milk and other dairy products, mushrooms, beef liver, as well as in supplements.

# Obesity

So, you attributed that belly fat to a mid-life crisis or hormonal challenge! Look at the pattern of sleep apnea, daytime sleepiness, and fatigue. Now think about your visceral obesity, insulin resistance, and other health issues! Is there a correlation? Could these factors be interconnected? We already know that obesity is a significant risk factor for sleep apnea. Some researchers believe that it is visceral fat, rather than generalized obesity, that predisposes people to the development of sleep apnea (Vgontzas et al., 2000).

But, how about if we think of obesity and fatigue as interrelated simply because we did not take the time for a decent, healthy meal? Perhaps we inhaled our fast food at the desk or nurse's station. Perhaps on your shift, there is no healthy food available to you, and you succumb to the snack bar or candy machine for a sugar high. This can clearly contribute to obesity, and when your weight is higher than normal, you can also suffer from increased fatigue. What might not tire someone else could very well tire you.

# CARDIOVASCULAR DISEASE

A lack of quality sleep can certainly contribute to high blood pressure and subsequent heart disease, but it can be a vicious circle. When you are persistently tired or chronically fatigued, you will be less healthy. Fatigue is a frequent sign of heart disease, especially in women.

If you have an existing cardiac problem, you are more likely to experience fatigue. Fatigue may be drug induced or lifestyle induced. Remember that fatigue is a symptom—something that is felt, such as a headache or dizziness. It is not a sign that can be detected on examination. So, know your body, report your symptoms, and be well.

What can you do to keep yourself heart healthy, fatigue-free, and feeling well? You can ensure adequate rest, hydration, nutrition, and exercise. You can make a concerted effort to take good care of your body so that your body will take good care of you.

*"When I'm tired, I rest. I say, 'I can't be a superwoman today.'"*

*—Jada Pinkett Smith*

# Fatigue Countermeasures

Fatigue countermeasures can be as simple as taking breaks. In patient care settings, per diem or float pool nurses can work during meal periods. Creative scheduling and nontraditional hours are an option for those who prefer to work partial shifts but want to remain active. A fatigue reduction management system (FRMS) is essential, regardless of the industry. There are several ways to structure an effective FRMS. One method was proposed by the American College of Occupational and Environmental Medicine (ACOEM) in their Guidance Statement on Fatigue Risk Management in the Workplace (ACOEM, 2012).

We can push our bodies and our minds just so far before they will fail us. Fatigue countermeasure programs should be offered by employers. In healthcare, they might include providing adequate staffing, ensuring breaks and meal periods, offering sleeping accommodations (such as a recliner and a timer), and establishing nap policies. The employee's responsibility is to obtain sufficient sleep prior to beginning a shift.

Institutional countermeasures include defining roles and responsibilities, training staff, assessing and reducing risk, defining performance indicators, and investigating sentinel events.

# Stakeholders

We all have a stake in the challenge; we are all the solution. Stakeholders are people or organizations that are invested in the program, are interested in the results of the evaluation, and/or have a stake in what will be done with the results of the evaluation. Representing their needs and interests throughout the process is fundamental to good program evaluation and to an effective countermeasure program.

In my field, which is health and well-being, the stakeholders are employers, policymakers, researchers, professional societies, caregivers, advocacy groups, providers, patients, and payers. Expectations may be high, and may differ substantially. However, we all want the same result: quality, safety, and good outcomes. By identifying and engaging those involved, we support collaboration.

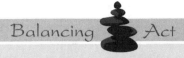

## RESOURCES

We are not alone, and there are multiple resources available regarding fatigue and combating it, including:

- National Sleep Foundation Patient Education Portal at www.sleepfoundation.org

- Nurse Fatigue—American Nurses Association at www. nursingworld.org/MainMenuCategories/WorkplaceSafety/ Healthy-Work-Environment/Work-Environment/NurseFatigue

- American Nurses Association Shift Work Sleep Disorder Kit at http://eo2.commpartners.com/users/swsd/

- Sleep and Sleep Disorders at www.cdc.gov/sleep

- Wisconsin Hospital Association, Inc. Fatigue and Hours of Work Toolkit at www.wha.org/fatigue.aspx

This chapter focused on fatigue and its impact on work, safety, well-being, and stress. Remember that stress is often manifested by emotional as well as physical symptoms, and we covered them all. You must assume responsibility for fatigue; it is not the work of the employer alone. Rather, steps that you take to maintain your own health, to avoid drowsiness and to be responsible, play a significant role in balance. And, this chapter examined those health issues like gastrointestinal, mood, depression, obesity, cardiovascular and more. Assuming a natural approach for health and wellness allows you to balance traditional allopathic methods with an integrative approach that considers the whole body and your behaviors.

The core issue here was fatigue; we all have a stake in the challenge; we are all the solution. We can find balance by knowing our body and its response to the stressors we face. We can find balance by taking steps to minimize fatigue.

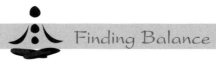

## Finding Balance

## REFLECTIONS

- Be aware of the symptoms of fatigue and take action.
- Assume responsibility for behaviors that will minimize fatigue.
- Take a natural approach to well-being.
- Use available resources to enhance your own knowledge base.

## REFERENCES

Agrawal, R., & Gomez-Pinilla, F. (2012). "Metabolic syndrome" in the brain: Deficiency in omega-3-fatty acid exacerbates dysfunctions in insulin receptor signaling and cognition. *The Journal of Physiology.* Retrieved by http://jp.physoc.org/content/early/2012/03/31/jphysiol.2012.230078.abstract

American College of Occupational and Environmental Medicine (ACOEM). (2012). Fatigue risk management in the workplace. *Journal of Occupational and Environmental Medicine, 54*(2), 231-258.

American Nurses Association (ANA). (2014a). Health & safety: Workplace fatigue. Retrieved from http://nursingworld.org/MainMenuCategories/WorkplaceSafety/Healthy-Work-Environment/Work-Environment/NurseFatigue

American Nurses Association (ANA). (2014b). Position paper on nurse fatigue.

Antunes, L. C., Levandovski, R., Dantas, G., Caumo, W., & Hidalgo, M. P. (2010). Obesity and shift work: Chronobiological aspects. *Nutrition Research Reviews, 23*(1), 155-168.

Bambra, C. L., Whitehead, M. M., Sowden, A. J., Akers, J., & Petticrew, M. P. (2008). A hard day's night? The effects of compressed working week interventions on the health and work-life balance of shift workers: A systematic review. *Journal of Epidemiology & Community Health, 62*(9), 764-777.

Barker, L. M., & Nussbaum, M. A. (2011). Fatigue, performance and the work environment: A survey of registered nurses. *Journal of Advanced Nursing, 67*(6), 1370-1382.

Borchard, T. (2011). Why sugar is dangerous to depression. PsychCentral. Retrieved from http://psychcentral.com/blog/archives/2011/07/13/why-sugar-is-dangerous-to-depression/

Brown, D. L., Feskanich, D., Sanchez, B. N., Rexrode, K. M., Schernhammer, E. S., & Lisabeth, L. D. (2010). Rotating night shift work and the risk of ischemic stroke. *American Journal of Epidemiology, 169*(11), 1370-1377.

Bushnell, P. T., Colombi, A., Caruso, C. C., & Tak, S. (2010). Work schedules and health behavior outcomes at a large manufacturer. *Industrial Health, 48*(4), 395-405.

Caldwell, J. A., Caldwell, J. L., Schmidt, R. M. (2008). Alertness management strategies for operational contexts. *Sleep Medicine Review, 12*(4), 257-273.

Dorrian, J., Lamond, N., Dawson, D. (2000). The ability to self-monitor performance when fatigued. *Journal of Sleep Research. 9*(2), 137-144.

Dorrian, J., Paterson, J., Pincombe, J., Grech, C., Rogers, A. E., & Dawson, D. (2011). Sleepiness, stress, and compensatory behaviors in nurses and midwives. *Revista de Saute Publica* (*Journal of Public Health*, Brazil), *45*(5), 922-930

Drake, D. A., Luna, M., Georges, J. M., & Steege, L. M. (2012). Hospital nurse force theory: A perspective of nurse fatigue and patient harm. *Advances in Nursing Science, 35*(4), 305-314.

Ernst, E. (2007). Herbal remedies for depression and anxiety. *Advances in Psychiatric Treatment, 13*, 312-316. Retrieved from http://apt.rcpsych.org/content/13/4/312.full

Hendren, R. (2011, May 17). How nurse executives can help tired nurses. Retrieved from www.healthleadersmedia.com/Page-1/NRS-266247/How-Nurse-Executives-Can-Help-Tired-Nurses

Holford, P. (2009). *The Low-GL Diet Bible.* London: Little, Brown Book Group.

Institute of Medicine (IOM). (2008). Resident duty hours: Enhancing sleep, supervision, and safety. Retrieved from http://iom.edu/-/media/Files/Report%20Files/2008/Resident-Duty-Hours/residency%20hours%20revised%20for%20web.pdf

The Joint Commission (TJC). (2011). Health care worker fatigue and patient safety. Sentinel Event Alert, 48. Retrieved from www.jointcommission.org/assets/1/18/sea_48.pdf

Khan A., Khan, S. R., Shankles, E. B., & Polissar, N. L. (2002). Relative sensitivity of the Montgomery-Asberg Depression Rating Scale, the Hamilton Depression rating scale and the Clinical Global Impressions rating scale in antidepressant clinical trials. *International Clinical Psychopharmacology, 17*(6), 281-285.

Lamond, N., & Dawson, D. (1999). Quantifying the performance impairment associated with fatigue. *Journal of Sleep Research, 8*(4), 255-262.

Lerman, S. E., Eskin, E., Flower, D. J., George, E. C., Gerson, B., Hartenbaum, N., & Moore-Ede, M. (2012). Fatigue risk management in the workplace. *Journal of Occupational and Environmental Medicine, 54*(2), 231-258.

Leung, A., Chan, C., Ng, J., and Wong, P. (2006). Factors contributing to officers' fatigue in speed maritime craft operations. *Applied Ergonomics, 37*(5), 565–576.

Lombardo, B., & Eyre, C. (2011). Compassion fatigue: A nurse's primer. *The Online Journal of Issues in Nursing, 16*(1). Retrieved from http://www.nursingworld. org/MainMenuCategories/ANAMarketplace/ANAPeriodicals/OJIN/ TableofContents/Vol-16-2011/No1-Jan-2011/Compassion-Fatigue-A-Nurses-Primer.html

Mayo Clinic Staff. (2014). Psychological fatigue. Mayo Clinic. Retrieved from http://www.mayoclinic.org/symptoms/fatigue/basics/definition/sym-20050894

National Highway Traffic Safety Administration (NHTSA). (2013). Early estimate of motor vehicle traffic fatalities in 2012. Traffic Safety Facts: Crash Stats. Retrieved from http://www-nrd.nhtsa.dot.gov/Pubs/811741.pdf

National Institutes of Health (NIH). (2014). Vitamin D: Fact sheet for consumer. Retrieved from http://ods.od.nih.gov/factsheets/VitaminD-QuickFacts/

Natural Prevention Council. (2011). National prevention strategy—America's plan for better health and wellness. Retrieved from http://www.surgeongeneral.gov/ initiatives/prevention/strategy/report.pdf

Nemets, B., Stahl, Z., & Belmaker, R. H. (2002). Addition of omega-3 fatty acid to maintenance medication treatment for recurrent unipolar depressive disorder. *American Journal of Psychiatry, 159*(3), 477-479.

Reed, K. (2013). Nursing fatigue and staffing costs: What's the connection? *Nursing Management, 44*(4), 47-50.

Rogers, A. E. (2012). Healthcare work schedules. In P. Carayon (Ed.), *Handbook of human factors and ergonomics in health care and patient safety* (pp. 199-208). New York: Taylor & Francis Group.

Smith, A., Sutherland, D., & Christopher, G. (2005). Effects of repeated doses of caffeine on mood and performance of alert and fatigued volunteers. *Journal of Psychopharmacology, 19*(6), 620-626.

Stoll, A., Severus, E., Freeman, M. P., Rueter, S., Zboyan, H. A., Diamond, E.,... Marangell, L. B. (1999). Omega 3 fatty acids in bipolar disorder: A preliminary double-blind, placebo-controlled trial. *Archives of General Psychiatry, 56*(5), 407-412. doi:10.1001/archpsyc.56.5.407.

Strawbridge, H. (2013). Going gluten-free just because? Here's what you need to know. Harvard Health Publications: Harvard Medical School. Retrieved from http://www.health.harvard.edu/blog/going-gluten-free-just-because-heres-what-you-need-to-know-201302205916

Turner, E. H., Loftis, J. M., & Blackwell, A. D. (2005). Serotonin a la carte: Supplementation with the serotonin precursor 5-hydroxytryptophan. *Pharmacology & Therapeutics.* http://www.academia.edu/280135/ Serotonin_a_la_carte_Supplementation_with_the_serotonin_precursor_5-hydroxytryptophan

Vgontzas, A. N., Papanicolaou, D. A., Bixler, E. O., Hopper, K., Lotsikas, A., Lin, H.,…Chrousos, G. P. (2000). Sleep apnea and daytime sleepiness and fatigue: Relation to visceral obesity, insulin resistance, and hypercytokinemia. *The Journal of Clinical Endocrinology and Metabolism. 85*(3), 1151-1155.

WebMD. (2013). Weakness and fatigue. Retrieved from http://www.webmd.com/ a-to-z-guides/weakness-and-fatigue-topic-overview

> "Life is like riding a bike. It is impossible to maintain your balance while standing still."
>
> —Linda Brakeall

# 8

# WORKPLACE BALANCE

*—Sharon M. Weinstein, MS, RN, CRNI, FACW, FAAN*

Good employers recognize the value of good employees and are often willing to find or create ways to help employees deal with family situations by making short-term or permanent changes in work schedules. Options include flextime, job-sharing, telecommuting, and part-time employment. If you know your skills, abilities, and performance record are strong and valued, you have a solid footing for negotiating flexible work arrangements.

## NEGOTIATION

What is negotiation? Practically, it's making the other person an offer or proposal that he or she may find more attractive than the next best alternative. Some consider negotiation to be the art of making deals. It is certainly that, but it also involves educating the other party about merits of your offer or proposal—or talents, skills, and actual and potential contributions. Negotiation is a key component of creating workplace balance and thus avoiding burnout. To negotiate successfully, you must do some advance planning. The process is simple, but each step is critical to the outcome.

1. Be prepared. Follow the tips and understand the rationale—know what you want and understand what the other party wants.

2. Open with your case; this demonstrates confidence. Then, listen actively.

3. Support your case with facts.

4. Explore areas of agreement and disagreement, and seek understanding and possibilities.

5. Indicate your readiness to work together.

6. Know your options.

7. Advance to closure by confirming the details.

8. Make it happen!

| Tip | Rationale |
| --- | --- |
| Know what you are willing to accept and be honest about your requirements. | You will be empowered in support of your interests. |
| | Your listener will recognize your confidence level. |
| Do not disclose what you are willing to accept in terms of salary or conditions. Have a deal-breaker in mind, e.g., lack of flexibility in hours. | This will compromise your negotiating power. |
| Determine what the other party is willing to accept. | It is better to know the alternatives up front than to second-guess. |
| Be an active listener, like a student. | Assume there are things about the situation that you don't understand. |
| | Let the other party know that you have heard and understood what has been said. |

# BURNOUT

If you are a busy person with a demanding job and family and friends who seek your time and attention, you are blessed, but *only* if you can handle it. Working from home can be beneficial, because you can maintain some control over your schedule.

*"To keep a lamp burning, we have to keep putting oil in it."*

*—Mother Teresa*

However, some busy people feel guilty regardless of what they are doing. They may feel guilty spending time with friends and family because they are not getting work done. Likewise, when working intensely, they feel guilty because they're not paying attention to others or taking good care of themselves. That feeling can lead to burnout—when the stress lasts so long that your ability to function is impaired. Dr. Audrey Canaff, on behalf of CareerBuilder (Lorenz, 2009), considers job burnout a response to work stress that leaves you feeling powerless and drained. Burnout symptoms include, but are not limited to:

- Powerlessness
- Hopelessness
- Emotional exhaustion
- Detachment
- Isolation
- Irritability

- Feeling trapped
- Failure
- Despair
- Cynicism
- Apathy

We hear a lot about burnout within the healthcare sector. Nurses work 12+ hour shifts and endure long stretches without time off. The demand on time and talent is extreme. When staffing is an issue, nurses work longer hours. When the economy is at an all-time low, nurses work additional hours or multiple jobs to make ends meet. This is true of many other industries as well.

Burnout can be prevented by following the advice of experts and those who have personally experienced burnout. The main point they make is that we benefit greatly by maintaining clear boundaries between our work lives and our personal lives.

# SETTING CLEAR BOUNDARIES

*"I arise in the morning torn between the desire to improve the world and a desire to enjoy the world. This makes it hard to plan the day."*

—E. B. White

When your work life and personal life blend together under the guise of "multitasking," both suffer. When you are at work, focus on the job to be done. When you are finished with work, don't bring it home with you. Make time for your personal life. If your work materials are dispersed throughout nearly every room of your house, you have no place for a real retreat. You're not spending high-quality time with friends or family members if you're talking on your cell phone or checking your email when you're with them. Take time to focus exclusively on your friends and family members when you're with them; then you won't feel guilty when you have to concentrate on work. Create high-quality work and personal experiences for yourself by keeping them separate.

## CREATE A DESIGNATED WORK AREA AT HOME

When you are in your home "office," that's the time to work, to respond to calls, complete electronic banking, update social media, and reply to email. When you are finished, walk away from the office and computer. Set aside specific times for checking messages. Then, reward yourself with personal time.

## MASTER EFFICIENCY

If you negotiate a telecommuting arrangement, keep in mind that many professionals find it difficult to adjust to working from home. The freedom of working in casual clothing, of not reporting for work at a specific time, and of not being directly supervised by others creates an environment that may become lax. You must be responsible for your own efficiency, effectiveness, and efforts. Is your work environment efficient and ergonomically correct? Does it lend itself to a high level of productivity in a short time span? Does your work schedule enable you to maximize your productivity? For example, are you a morning person—someone who works best in the early hours of the day? Set a schedule to plan your work at home, and then work according to your plan.

## MANAGE YOUR TIME WISELY

You schedule appointments with other people in your personal planner, so why not schedule time with yourself? Make appointments for regular exercise, a hearty walk, or meditation. Regardless of whom you are and what you do, you still have the same 24 hours in each day. Do you delegate, or are you the one who must do it all to get it right?

When you are in a meeting with others, be engaged. Do not check your mobile phone for messages; leave it in your purse, briefcase, or pocket. Interruptions are bound to occur during the day; think about how you handle them, and how you return to the task at hand. It is sometimes good to leave small blocks of time throughout the day for flexible scheduling and unplanned activities. The schedule is a protective shield; it keeps you from overwhelming yourself, so use it wisely.

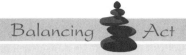

## IF YOU MISS AN APPOINTMENT WITH YOURSELF...

If you find that you don't have the discipline to keep the appointment with yourself, include a friend or family member in the healthy activity and make an appointment with them. It will be harder to postpone, and you'll have quality time with that person as a bonus.

## KNOW WHAT IS IMPORTANT AND WHY

In his book *The 7 Habits of Highly Effective People* (2004), Stephen Covey showed that for many of us, the day is filled with tasks that attract our attention and seem urgent, but they may never need to be done. Weed those out and make time for the important tasks. The important duties that are also urgent require our immediate attention. Learn to prioritize. Know that the things you must complete today, or this week, are most important, and engage in systems that can help you to stick to your schedule.

## KNOW YOUR LIMITATIONS

Are you an assertive type who finds it easy to say "no"? Or, are you a self-less type who takes on more than you can possibly handle? Negotiate for workplace balance by knowing yourself and your limitations, and remember that "no" can be a complete sentence. This means that it's perfectly acceptable to say "no" without any further explanation. Nurses are notorious for putting the needs of others before their own. Perhaps part of the gratification nurses get from their job is being of service to others. To effectively care for others, you must center yourself. There are several centering techniques. Many involve being quiet and still with yourself—either sitting, walking, or absorbed in a hobby. You can find one that works for you. Practice your technique even when you feel great. It will help prevent stress and burnout.

## CENTERING YOURSELF

Leonard Orr originated a technique called conscious breathing that you can use to help center yourself. You can access information on Orr's approach (20 Connected Breaths) from http://rebirthingbreathwork.com/2013/03/16/555/

## RECOGNIZE THE NEED FOR HELP

In today's work environment, there are multiple options available to employees, including employee assistance programs (EAPs). These are employer or group-supported programs designed to alleviate personal and workplace issues. A comprehensive program can add value to staff and management. The U.S. Department of Labor's Office of Disability Employment Policy (2009) defines EAP services as follows:

| Employees and Family Members | Organizations |
| --- | --- |
| Mental health-related services and referrals | Educational programs on managing mental health, stress, and addictions in the workplace |
| Drug and alcohol-related services and referrals | Safety and emergency preparedness |
| Referrals for personal issues | Communications related to mergers, layoffs, death |
| Wellness and health promotion | Smoking cessation programs and weight reduction groups |

ComPsych is the world's largest provider of employee assistance programs addressing behavioral health, wellness, work-life, absence management and more (ComPsych, 2014).

## SEEK HELP

Successful people are not afraid to ask for help. Everyone needs help from time to time, and reaching out is an admirable skill. Be acutely aware of the stressors in your schedule and in your life. Know thyself first! Manage yourself, and take advantage of counseling, coaches, professional peers, and mentors. Winston Churchill said that a laborer benefits from physical rest and a sedentary person benefits from exercise. Those of us who deal with people can benefit by switching to an activity that absorbs the mind and makes it difficult to think about our problems for a while.

## COMMUNICATE NEEDS CLEARLY

If there is a teenager in your house, you fully understand the concepts of perception and reception. It is like the game known as "Telephone" or "Whispering Down the Lane." What you said is not always what is heard. Maintain a positive attitude and be clear in your statement. Make a connection with your listener, whether your communication is verbal or written. Request feedback.

### Action Item
### LISTENING STRATEGIES

Communication is a two-way process; it can improve employee engagement, workplace morale, and productivity. Here are some tips:

1. Pay attention by looking directly at the speaker and avoid side conversations.

2. Demonstrate that you are listening by nodding occasionally and encouraging the speaker to continue with comments like "yes."

3. Offer feedback by paraphrasing what has been said.

4. Respond appropriately and respectfully.

5. Be positive and team-centered.

When I worked in the new independent states of the former Soviet Union, I had the privilege of mentoring the next generation of nurse leaders. We often played "Whispering down the Lane" to communicate a thought. Imagine having 35 emerging nurse leaders in the room who spoke at least one of five languages. The reinterpretation of what was said was comical, but it reinforced the concept of clear communication.

## MEASURE YOUR OUTCOMES

If the primary source of communication is online, you can easily measure outcomes by views, followers, engagement, and conversation. You will know and understand your impact. A goal is needed to measure that outcome. In today's environment, a department store can measure how much time you spend at the cosmetics counter or in the shoe department, and they do it electronically. Your utility company can monitor your utilization electronically; unfortunately, this process can also contribute to poor health (see Chapter 6 on the effects of technology.)

At the end of the day, you want to know you've been successful and that you have achieved something. I worked in Europe, on United States Agency for International Development (USAID) programs, and the government wanted to measure outputs. In our structure, that meant evaluating the number of visitors to hospital sites in the United States and abroad, the number of professional and technical exchanges, and expectations. The most effective way to measure outcomes, as opposed to outputs, is to determine impact, leads generated, or resources used more efficiently.

## MEASURING OUTCOMES

1. Aim for relevant outcomes—those that you can demonstrate.

2. Plan the evaluation mechanism and programs concurrently.

3. Identify baseline status.

4. Use existing research; most nonprofits use data that has been demonstrated in the past.

5. Use predictors or intended outcomes to demonstrate impact; diet, exercise and lifestyle could be predictors of health.

6. When funding is being sought, focus on what matters to the funding organization.

## TEND TO YOUR OWN INTERESTS

Tending to your own interests is not the same thing as minding your own business. Instead, it refers to the fact that you should be free to explore your own interests and outlets—those things that bring you joy. Complete yourself by being whole, being on purpose, and being intentional.

## TRY SOMETHING NEW

You may know that what you are doing now is not working well. Perhaps the balance between your work and personal life is off. Working harder at the same activities does not create balance. Consider changing your schedule or altering your routine to try to reset the balance. Exercise in the morning instead of after work. Find a combination that works best for you and that reenergizes your life.

In their book *Just Enough* (2004), Laura Nash and Howard Stevenson showed through in-depth interviews, case studies, and surveys of top executives that successful people who found the greatest satisfaction in their lives paid attention to happiness, achievement, significance, and legacy throughout their entire lives. Nash and Stevenson recommend that we continually seek contentment and accomplishment, and that we focus on making a positive impact on people we care about and ways to help others find future success. We can do these things, and prevent burnout at the same time, by being mindful of how we're living moment to moment.

An important element of preventing burnout is the actual work environment. Whether we work independently or as members of a team, people can and do make the difference!

# HAVE THE RIGHT PEOPLE IN THE RIGHT SEATS ON THE BUS

*"Whoever is happy will make others happy too."*

*—Anne Frank*

Having a lot of help is not enough if it isn't the right help for the right job. Make a concerted effort to surround yourself with good people, and give them the latitude they need to do a good job. As an example, within the nursing community, having the right people in a busy emergency department (ED) ensures appropriate triage, timely service, and quality outcomes. Because there is no such thing as the "average" day in the ED, members of the healthcare team can collectively:

- Define stretch targets for length of stay.
- Implement a monitoring system for status of patients in emergency departments to be reviewed at predefined intervals.
- Coordinate resources.
- See the right person at the right time.
- Fast-track patients as needed.
- Track communications with patients who are
  - Waiting to be seen
  - Waiting for admission
  - Waiting for discharge

Another good example is from an Institute for Healthcare Improvement (IHI) (2008) initiative developed by The Florida Hospital, Orlando, Florida, team whose goal was to decrease door-to-door time in the emergency department.

The team, with the right key players in place, implemented the following strategic actions:

- **Predictive model:** They looked at the previous 4 weeks of volume, key metrics, and admissions and determined daily demand. Staffing is consistent with demand.

- **Lab turnaround:** They decreased time in getting specimens to the lab, thus facilitating receipt of results.

- **Efficiency:** They looked for and decreased wasted or non-value-added steps. They observed and videotaped processes and redesigned work areas to ensure closer proximity to patients.

- **Tools:** They incorporated lean tools into daily process. Some of the tools are single patient flow and simplifying tasks.

- **Process council:** They developed a monthly process council. Representation includes nursing and senior leadership. Following process review and outcomes, action plans are developed to help the team meet its goals.

You can easily apply examples like these to your clinical setting; they contribute to positive outcomes, staff satisfaction, and balance.

Working as a team, you and your colleagues can achieve successes unattainable by lone individuals. The knowledge that there are others around you who are pulling with you to attain a shared goal enhances the rewards of a professional nursing career.

## TEAM BENEFITS

Football, soccer, and baseball are team sports, and they all require that the team work together to be successful. If you are a part of a team, but you function like the Lone Ranger rather than the Brady Bunch, the team will suffer, and so will the outcomes. Teams in business environments can achieve far more than the sum of the individual skills alone. Consider these benefits:

- They can generate a wider range of ideas.
- They are self-motivated.
- They can brainstorm.
- They often take more risks than individuals.
- They have a range of personalities and styles such as workers, thinkers, leaders who contribute the right balance of skills necessary to achieve high performance.
- They support each other.
- They provide mentoring.

Think about the high-performing teams with which you have worked and identify the aspects of teamwork that are, or were, most beneficial.

## TEAM INTEGRATION

The team may become a unit due to an organizational restructure, a merger or acquisition, or an institutional change. When a company I represented merged with two similar companies with very different corporate cultures, attention was given to how the teams would integrate. What would happen when there could be only one vice president of operations within the new model, eliminating two highly skilled professionals from the picture?

Think about how you transition others out of the work environment and welcome new employees in a nonthreatening way. There are lots of things that your new team member needs to know to start adding value to the team. Be sure to provide context, including the team's mandate, your strategy, the goals and objectives, and any other formal documents that will help the person understand what you're trying to achieve. This is often overlooked.

## INTEGRATION STRATEGIES

1. Welcome the newcomer prior to the first day

2. Plan specific orientation activities including meetings with key personnel and workgroups

3. Allocate assigned workspace and ensure comfort with the environment

4. Add the newcomer to relevant mail distribution lists

5. Provide orientation manuals and training

6. Orient the newcomer to the IT systems and services

7. Prepare a calendar for the first month of meetings and activities

8. Provide guidance regarding available resources

## LEVERAGE YOUR TEAM

An outstanding example of leverage may be found in the network marketing model of business (King & Robinson, 2013). John Paul Getty once said, "I would rather earn 1% of 100 people's efforts than 100% of my own efforts." Network marketing, as a business model, creates teams that leverage the efforts of others. The result of the efforts of thousands is the generation of residual income. Think about it—the Disney family continues to earn from the work of their patriarch. The Sinatra family continues to earn from the early works of the late Frank Sinatra. And book authors earn residual income on the books sold. Residual income is created through leverage.

Imagine that you are in the business of mowing lawns and that you could earn $40 per lawn. If you were to average five lawns per day, you would earn a gross income of $200 a day before expenses. This is an example of a linear income where you use 100% of your own efforts to create an income. This is what the majority of people do their entire lives.

Now imagine that you owned a lawn mowing referral business where instead of mowing the lawns yourself, you work "on" your business, rather than "in" it. You spend your time finding lawns that need to be mowed and employ contractors to do the physical work. Suppose that you now employ 20 contractors, each of whom mows five lawns per day. You pay each contractor $30 per lawn, but you charge $40, earning a profit of $10 per lawn. Do the math—you are now mowing 100 lawns a day, which you could not have done alone. You are leveraging the skills of others to achieve your goals.

In healthcare, perhaps you serve as a health coach. Rather than coach each client yourself, you create a team of health coaches who have similar credentials. Perhaps they are strategically positioned nationwide, and because they have aligned themselves with you and your coaching organization, you receive residual income on their efforts as well as your own.

## Allow Others to Connect with You

Today, we have to be concerned about our kids' connections online while they are playing games or interacting. Although we used to know all of their friends, that might no longer be true. Some of their contacts may be remote; the same is true for your own contacts.

Be open to meeting new people, to connecting with others in your workplace and beyond. Meet with others for tea or coffee to share ideas, challenges, or opportunities. Remember that there are no problems in the workplace—just opportunities for improvement. Much of that occurs when you connect with others and look at a bigger picture of what is possible. Enrich yourself by reaching out!

# Family-Friendly Work Environments

Family-friendly working and work/life balance refer to working arrangements that help us achieve a better balance between work and family life. These may include maternity and paternity leave, on-site child care, flextime, job sharing, working from home, and other creative solutions. They all add value to the work environment, and they contribute to workplace balance.

*"When people go to work, they shouldn't have to leave their hearts at home."*

—Betty Bender

## Reentering the Workforce

If you are reentering the workforce after taking time off, your preference may be to work part time or have a flexible schedule. If your priorities in life require that you have a flexible work schedule or work part-time, you should inform a potential employer of those expectations during the interview process. Otherwise, you may be dissatisfied with the working conditions and be unable to handle the stress at work and at home. Job hopping can be stressful, and changing positions may not be possible when the economy is poor. See Chapter 11 for more information.

## Switching to Part-Time Work

Ideally, switching to part-time employment should not be a challenge. You may, however, want to consider working some from home to demonstrate your credibility and efficiency. As discussions continue, your track record of excellence could work in your favor.

Negotiate based on a specific project. If your current assignment requires skill sets that only you can provide, negotiate your time and availability accordingly. Demonstrate your flexibility by continuing on a full-time basis until the project is underway and then renegotiate a part-time schedule in your favor.

If your goal is to work part time, consider the following:

- How many hours can you take off without affecting your benefits?
- Would your manager be supportive of the situation? If not, could you be more flexible?

## WORK/LIFE BALANCE

We all have responsibilities, whether caring for children or elderly parents, or pursuing personal interests, activities, or hobbies. Some of us are in the "sandwich generation," meaning that we're juggling the challenge of school-age children and aging parents or family members. Workers must be equipped to resolve personal and workplace issues, juggle conflicting responsibilities, and balance personal and workplace roles.

*"We need to maintain a proper balance in our life by allocating the time we have. There are occasions where saying no is the best time management practice there is."*

*—Catherine Pulsife*

At the same time, today's employers are constantly seeking ways to assist their workers in managing their job responsibilities and their personal responsibilities and needs. Strategies for work/life balance help create supportive, healthy work environments; strengthen employee commitment and loyalty; and result in more productive workplaces and improved customer satisfaction.

As clinicians, we entered the field of nursing with a common goal—caring for, and about, others and providing the best possible outcomes. As professionals, we also have expectations from our work environment, from those with whom we work, and our future. If your path is paved with good intentions, but your work is unrewarding and your time is not your own, negotiate. Think things over and make a change.

*"Right now you are one choice away from a new beginning—one that leads you toward becoming the fullest human being you can be."*

*—Oprah Winfrey*

# Tip the Scales in Your Favor

Many of us are working harder than ever before. Our hours and days are longer. Our free time is nominal. We lack free time, even at home, because there is too much to do and life gets in the way. We may have fallen into the technology trap because—after all—it is available 24/7. Take a look at your own situation and be honest with yourself. What is in your way? Could you possibly be getting in your own way? You can tip the scales in your favor with the addition of counterbalancing techniques like time management, prioritization, health awareness, and openness.

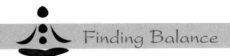

Finding Balance

### Find Focus

For one day, notice how often you are not focusing on the task at hand. For example, during a phone call, are you thinking of what you have to do after you are done with the call? Are you straightening the clutter on your desk as you listen to a coworker?

Before you make a call or keep an appointment, take a moment beforehand to say to yourself, "I will give this my full attention." Then do it.

### Track Your Time

Do you often find yourself at the end of the day wondering where the time went? Consider tracking how long it takes you to do routine tasks so that you can better plan your time.

### Make an Appointment

Right now, make an appointment for lunch or another activity with a friend or relative you have been meaning to spend time with.

## BECOME A NETWEAVER

Littell (2003) coined the concept of NetWeaving, a form of networking that focuses on helping others instead of the "what's in it for me" concept of networking. Apply NetWeaving in your work and home life:

1. Take the time to make at least one connection between two people who can help each other, knowing that good deeds often reward the person doing them.

2. Identify one way you can share your expertise with others. It might be as simple as agreeing to share examples of reports you have written to someone who has never done one.

*Source: http://www.netweaving.com/*

## REFLECTIONS

- No one knows you better than you; work that to your advantage.

- Become a master of efficiency.

- Identify those areas of life most important for your well-being and balance and integrate them within your lifestyle.

- Know your limits.

- Treat yourself with kindness.

## REFERENCES

ComPsych. (2014). About ComPsych. Retrieved from http://www.compsych.com/about

Covey, S. (2004). *The 7 habits of highly effective people.* New York: Simon and Schuster, Inc. (Free Press Division).

Institute for Healthcare Improvement (IHI). (2008). Reducing ED door-to-doctor time by implementing lean process and tools. Retrieved from http://www.ihi.org/resources/Pages/ImprovementStories/ReducingDoortoDoctorTimebyImplementingLeanProcessandTools.aspx

King, C., & Robinson, J. (2013). *The New Professionals: The Rise of Network Marketing as the Next Major Profession.* Roseville, CA: Prima Publishing.

Littell, R. (2003). The heart and art of NetWeaving: Building meaningful relationships one connection at a time. Netweaving International Press. Retrieved from http://www.netweaving.com/index.php/books/

Lorenz, K. (2009). 5 signs of job burnout…and what to do about it. CareerBuilder. http://www.careerbuilder.com/Article/CB-655-The-Workplace-5-Signs-of-Job-Burnout-and-What-to-Do-About

Nash, L., & Stevenson, H. (2004). *Just enough: Tools for creating success in your work and life.* New York, NY: John Wiley & Sons.

Orr, L. (2013) 20 connected breaths—sets of 4 short, 1 long. Rebirthing Breathwork International. http://rebirthingbreathwork.com/2013/03/16/555/

U.S. Department of Labor. (2009). Employee assistance programs for a new generation of employees: Defining the next generation. Office of Disability Employment Policy. Retrieved from http://www.dol.gov/odep/documents/employeeassistance.pdf

"Laugh and the world laughs with you, snore and you sleep alone."

—Anthony Burgess

# 9

# SLEEPLESS, AND NOT JUST IN SEATTLE

*—Sharon M. Weinstein, MS, RN, CRNI, FACW, FAAN*

Sleep deficits contribute to poor health, chronic disease, and more. We are sleepless, not just in Seattle but across the country and around the world. Sleep is one of the most important components of a healthy lifestyle. The Centers for Disease Control and Prevention (CDC, n.d.) refers to insufficient sleep as a public health epidemic and links lack of sleep to automotive accidents, occupational errors, health issues, and more (CDC, n.d.; U.S. Department of Transportation [USDOT], n.d.). Insufficient sleep refers to the quality as well as the quantity of sleep.

If you do not make conscious choices about your habits for nourishing and restoring yourself, chances are that you may not actually be getting the kind of sleep that is nourishing or restoring you. Any choice that gives you less than what is for your greatest good is a choice that is going to deplete your storehouse of energy reserves and health; tax all the functions, organs, and cells of your body; and gradually impair your well-being. Sleep is one of the most significant factors in achieving mental and physical well-being.

# THE SLEEP CYCLE

For every living organism, there is a sleep cycle. A healthy day follows a natural cycle—one that allows the body to be rested. When you rest, you should be completely relaxed. This means you shouldn't be doing any mental work so that the mind and brain can simply recover. The pure "science" includes meditation or self-reflection (see Chapter 5), which promotes peace, tranquility, and balance. Deepak Chopra (n.d.) states that restful sleep provides the foundation for your mental and physical well-being.

*"My father said there were two kinds of people in the world: givers and takers. The takers may eat better, but the givers sleep better."*

*–Marlo Thomas*

Do you awaken with a spring in your step, ready to face the day with joy? Or, do you awaken to the sound of an alarm that triggers anxiety because of a deficit in your sleep cycle? There are two main types of sleep—non-rapid eye movement (NREM) sleep also known as quiet sleep, and rapid eye movement (REM) sleep, also known as active or paradoxical sleep. Within these two types are various phases, known as the four stages of sleep. Let's examine them here.

## RAPID EYE MOVEMENT AND THE STAGES OF SLEEP

As we sleep, we pass through different stages of sleep (Cherry, n.d.).

- **Stage 1**—In Stage 1, we experience light sleep, also known as Alpha. We are between being awake and entering sleep.
- **Stage 2**—Stage 2 occurs at the onset of sleep. We are becoming disengaged with the environment; our breathing and heart rate are regular, and our body temperature decreases. This is the Drowsy phase.

- **Stages 3 and 4**—Stages 3 and 4 are the deepest and most restorative sleep; they are also known as Delta phases. Our blood pressure drops; breathing is slower; energy is regained; and hormones are released for growth and development.

REM sleep (or paradoxical sleep) first occurs about 90 minutes after we fall asleep and increases over the later part of night. It is needed to provide energy to the brain and body. We are in REM sleep state for about 25% of the night. During this phase, the brain is active and dreams occur; our eyes dart back and forth during this stage. Our bodies become immobile and relaxed; our muscles shut down; and breathing and heart rate may become irregular. REM sleep is important to daytime performance and may contribute to memory enhancement (National Institute of Neurological Disorders and Stroke, n.d.).

## CIRCADIAN RHYTHM

The circadian rhythm plays a key role in the energy involved in all metabolic functions. Our circadian rhythm is interrupted when sleep is interrupted (American Academy of Sleep Medicine, 2008; National Institute of General Medical Sciences, n.d.). When we do shift work we often experience disturbances in our circadian rhythms. Much has been written about shift work disorders and the impact disruptions can have on the human body at the cellular level. So after a long flight, repeated shift work, or other changes in our normal sleep cycle, how do we reset the clock? Refer to "Workplace Stress" in Chapter 3.

## SIGNS OF DEPRIVATION

If you work in patient care you have possibly witnessed sleep deprivation in the critical-care units. For example, the patient comes to the hospital and expects to rest, but rest rarely comes easily simply because of the plethora of procedures that must be done and vital signs that must be checked. Think about trying to sleep amid noise, alarms, discomfort, and stress. Think of how your body responds to stressors in our environment, and how that affects your sleep process. The signs of deprivation include feeling tired or drowsy at any time throughout the day and having the ability to fall asleep within 5 minutes of lying down. Other symptoms include inability to handle stress, decreased memory, lack of concentration, increased appetite, poor decision-making skills, visual problems, and diminished motor skills.

*"The night is the hardest time to be alive and 4am knows all my secrets."*

—Poppy Z. Brite

## Recharging Your Batteries

We spend one-third of our lives in bed, yet we are sleep deprived. We need to recharge our batteries, and the best way to make that happen is to ensure a decent night's sleep. Every living being must sleep, at one time or another.

You recharge your mobile phone, your tablet, and other devices when the batteries run down. You accomplish this by simply plugging them in. After a little time—*voilà*—they are ready to go, full of energy and operating full steam ahead. We charge them because we know that they will not function without full power. But what about recharging your batteries so that you have enough power?

### Your Most Valuable Commodity

The human body is your most vulnerable commodity, and it needs—actually, it must have—sleep in order to recharge. We now know that deep sleep (stages 3 and 4) appears to be the most physically restorative sleep. Growth hormone is emitted during deep sleep, and this is the hormone that, among other things, tells tissue to repair itself after a long day of possible damage. In addition, growth hormone tells our bodies how to store fat, and where to put it. Most of your morning energy is dependent upon the amount of deep sleep that you get.

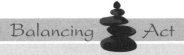

## HEALTH BENEFITS OF SLEEP

Sleep is a basic necessity of life, as important to our health and well-being as air, food, and water. When we sleep well, we wake up feeling refreshed, alert, and ready to face daily challenges. When we don't sleep well, every part of our lives can suffer. Our jobs, relationships, productivity, health, and safety (and that of those around us) are put at risk. Lack of sleep is taking a serious toll on our health, productivity, and lives.

*"The amount of sleep required by the average person is 5 minutes more."*

—Wilson Mizener

## HOW MUCH IS TOO MUCH?

We all know what is right for us. We know our bodies much better than anyone else. How much sleep do we really need? What is right for one person may not work for another. Take a look at the numbers and see if you are getting the right number of sleep hours for your own body. I think back to when my third child was born; it seemed as if she never took a nap after 6 months of age, because as child number 3, she was afraid to miss something.

The following are the recommended number of hours of sleep according to The Mayo Clinic (Morgenthaler, 2013).

Adults (18+): 7 to 8 hours

Teens (11-17): 8.5 to 9.5 hours

School-Age Children (5-10 years): 9 to 11 hours

Preschoolers (3-5 years): 11 to 13 hours

Toddlers (1-3 years): 12 to 14 hours (including naps)

Infants (3-11 months): 14 to 15 hours (including naps)

Newborns (0-2 months): 12 to 18 hours

# SHIFT WORK DISORDERS/DEFICITS

With around-the-clock lifestyles, our 24/7 society can keep us from allocating enough time for sleep or can put us on irregular schedules. When exactly did 24/7 become a way of life? Did it start with 2:00 a.m. feedings or the connectivity to our work? Feeling sleepy is a common experience, particularly for more than 20 million American shift workers. The body never quite adjusts to shift work!

When my children were young, I worked nights (the pay was higher), and I had problems staying awake long enough in the morning to get the kids to school. Sometimes I would "just rest" on the sofa and be sound asleep in minutes. Perhaps you have experienced something similar.

Working nontraditional schedules is a risk for on-the-job accidents and motor vehicle accidents. It is often difficult to get quality sleep during the day and support from others is important. To help themselves adapt, shift workers can perform a bedroom makeover, including making changes to music and lighting (see the tips in the "Your Sleep Environment" section later in the chapter). Be sure that the room is not too warm; lower temperatures tell your body that it is time for sleep, regardless of the actual time of day.

*"But I have promises to keep, and miles to go before I
sleep, and miles to go before I sleep."*

–Robert Frost

## PERFORMANCE DEFICITS

Can lack of sleep affect performance? We now recognize that insufficient
sleep is associated with poor attention and performance deficits (Mullington, Haack, Toth, Serrador, & Meier-Ewert, 2009). We often hear about
the ramifications of being tired and how it affects performance. An Ohio
man whose wife died in an automobile accident sued the hospital in a
wrongful death suit, claiming that she was "worked to death" and that the
hospital was aware of it (Allnurses, 2013). Staff shortages in the healthcare
and other industries are a nationwide issue. A good night's sleep sets the
stage for physical and mental performance.

## CATCHING UP

Recovering from a sleep deficit accumulated over five nights requires more
than one weekend night of sleeping longer. If you have young children in
the home, there is not much chance of sleeping beyond 7:00 a.m. on weekends. Very few people can manage with 4 or 5 hours of sleep, although they
often say that they can still function. The "work warriors" who do more, do
it better, and work on overdrive often state that they don't need 8 hours of
sleep, but chances are that they do. When a deficit has been established, it is
difficult to catch up.

## SLEEP MORE AND AGE LESS

We hear it all of the time—age matters! Nowhere is this truer than when
we discuss the sleep cycle in relation to midlife women. Sleep problems affect midlife women as they approach and pass through menopause at rates
higher than during other stages of life (Shaver & Zenk, 2000). Obesity,
hypertension, snoring, daytime headaches, and daytime sleepiness may
also exacerbate sleep problems (Albuquerque, Hachul, Andersen, & Tufik,
2014).

Assess the quality of your sleep by using the following tool; give yourself the number of points before each statement:

*Quantity of sleep*

(3) I make time for a good night's sleep

(2) I try to make time for a good night's sleep

(1) I get a good night's sleep when I can fit it in

*Quality of sleep*

(3) I awaken refreshed

(2) I have trouble falling asleep

(1) I take medications to fall asleep

*Daytime alertness*

(3) I remain alert throughout the day

(2) I sometimes wish that I could take a nap

(1) I never feel truly awake

*Age-related factors*

(3) I sleep as well now as I ever did

(2) I don't know what has happened to me

(1) Lack of sleep affects my memory

A score of 10 to 12 indicates that you rest easily and are a great sleeper. Keep it up for a lifetime. A score of 7 to 9 means that you need to focus on the need for sleep. A score of 4 to 6 indicates a detriment to longevity and health. A score less than 4 spells trouble.

# Your Sleep Environment

We know that a healing environment contributes to a healthy workplace, a healthy home, and a healthy body. Our sleep environment says much about our sleep patterns. For example, if you have a teenager who sleeps with a mobile phone under her pillow because she is afraid to miss a text, she is resting in a very unhealthy environment. Take whatever steps are needed to ensure that your environment is restful and conducive to a good night's sleep.

## Music

Soft music contributes to sound sleep. Think about the lullabies you may have used to soothe a fussy baby, or the song that you played for a toddler to suggest sleep. Music has healing properties. Listening to peaceful, sedative music at bedtime may be the most effective and inexpensive way to improve your sleep. Of course, the type of music matters. Rap and rock do not constitute restful music.

## Lighting

Soft, soothing lights help enhance the environment. Have you ever fallen asleep with the lights on and the TV blaring? Do you use your computer just before going to bed? Exposure to light stimulates a nerve pathway from the eye to parts of the brain that control hormones, body temperature, and other functions essential to a good night's sleep. Regulating your exposure to light is a good way to keep the circadian rhythms in check. Start the control process about an hour before going to bed—then it's lights out!

## Sound

Sound machines, also called white noise machines, have found their way into the bedroom; they emit an array of tranquil sounds like rain, wind, and birds chirping. If you live in a high traffic area where the sounds of passing cars last throughout the night, or if you live near railroad tracks, a sound machine will make all of the difference in the world. This device also drowns out sounds of snoring from a sleep companion—human or animal.

## MONITORS

Perhaps you have used an infant monitor to keep track of a newborn baby or young child. Monitors and other devices emit electromagnetic fields that compromise the sleep process and long-term health. Most baby monitors are now wireless, and this is the type that can cause damage. If you must have a monitor, use a corded (analog) monitor. Analog monitors only have a few channels, but even they should be kept 3 feet or more from the child's bed. Take care to remove the microwave radiation from your child's room to protect the developing brain; this will give everyone a better night's sleep.

## DEVICES

I have purchased any device that I thought might minimize my husband's snoring (although he denies ever snoring). I bought nose clips, nose tape, and any other noninvasive device I could find. Sleep medicine is big business, and the number of tools and gadgets continues to proliferate. Sleep monitors, continuous positive airway pressure (CPAP) devices, and other tools are promoted to eliminate sleep apnea. You should always consult your healthcare provider before you begin using any device.

Some of these gadgets, like phone apps that monitor sleep, actually interfere with the sleep cycle. Devices like cell phones and tablets should not be charged in the bedroom. Power strips should be removed from under the bed.

# LIFE IN THE WAY

Life does, and will get in the way. Life is bound to throw you a few curveballs. What do you do when the unexpected comes crashing into your world? Your palms sweat and your heart races. You think, "How did this happen?" And you can be certain that your sleep will be impaired during these tough times. Perhaps it is time to rethink your schedule and identify those things that you can eliminate so that you will be less stressed (see Chapter 2).

How many things are on your schedule right now that you wish would disappear? Why do you say yes when every fiber in your body is screaming no? How can you stave off the "Yes, Of Course" Syndrome to keep from feeling drained? How can you ensure that you take time for yourself so that your body will take care of you? Don't let life get in the way of living and of sleeping!

# Sleep Tools

Quality of sleep is a function of the tools you use as much as it is a function of the sleep process. The mattress, pillow, and other sleep accessories contribute to, or deter from, your sleep experience.

## Impact of the Mattress

Although there are many specialty mattresses available, the age of the mattress is also a key factor in restful sleep. A newer mattress (1 to 4 years of age) is thought to produce more optimal sleep. Most mattresses come with a manufacturer's warranty for 10, 15, or perhaps 20 years; that only refers to the materials and not the structure or support.

## A Simple, Yet Functional, Pillow

Sometimes I think that I will buy anything. Over the years I have purchased numerous pillows, each of which promised comfort, a good night's sleep, and proper neck support. I've bought molded pillows, magnetic pillows, anti-snoring pillows, and foam pillows. The right pillow can make the difference between waking up refreshed from a good night's sleep and waking up bleary-eyed with a sore back and a stiff neck. I now sleep on a silk pillow, and I love it. Decide what works best for you and then sleep on it.

## SLEEP MASKS AND LINENS

High-quality linens and a sleep mask can certainly enhance the sleep process. I have also spent a fortune on what one might consider high-quality linens over the years; although they were high cost, they were not always high in sleep value. I have found that the eco-functional bedding that I now use has properties that support the sleep process, and it is economical as well. The properties are infused within each fiber; consequently, the sheets can be machine washed and dried more than 10,000 times and still have the beneficial properties. This is different than children's sleepwear, which is generally coated with fire-retardant properties. When the sleepwear is washed and dried, it no longer retains those values. Properties that support the sleep process include chitin, bamboo charcoal, far-infrared, and negative ions (Alphay, n.d.).

| | |
|---|---|
| **Chitin** | Anti-mite |
| | Anti-bacterial |
| | Absorbs humidity |
| **Bamboo Charcoal** | Promotes circulation |
| | Absorbs and emits infrared rays |
| | Controls body temperature and humidity |
| | Deodorizes |
| | Releases negative ions |
| **Far-Infrared** | Controls body temperature |
| | Promotes circulation |
| | Absorbs moisture |
| **Negative Ions** | Supports immunity |
| | Boosts energy |
| | Increases oxygen to the brain |
| | Lifts mood and improves metabolism |

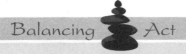

## SLEEP POSITIONS

Back, front, side—how should one sleep and what is best for the body, mind, and spirit?

Sleeping on the back aligns the head, neck, and spine in a neutral position. It is thought to lessen acid reflux, and it does not contribute to facial wrinkling. On the downside, if one has sleep apnea, snores, or is pregnant, pressure on the airway increases and could create discomfort. In later months of pregnancy, avoid sleeping on the back to keep the weight of the growing fetus off of the intestines and major blood vessels.

Sleeping on the side elongates the spine and helps to ease back pain. It could also prevent snoring, but it puts uneven weight on the neck and shoulder.

Sleeping on the stomach forces the spine out of its natural S-curve alignment and may generate pain, numbness, and tingling.

# BATTLING SLEEP DEPRIVATION AND MINIMIZING DISTURBANCES

Cellular metabolism and utilization of the nutrients consumed requires the proper quality sleep. The two are synergistic and enhance each other. As a culture, we are experiencing a dramatic increase in sleep deprivation and disturbances.

Most bedrooms now have TVs, sound systems, computers, phones, and alarm clocks. They are no longer just a place for sleep. This is true of even children's rooms. Unfortunately, these units, such as the baby monitor, emit electromagnetic frequencies (EMFs) that are disruptive to the human energy system—sometimes seriously so. Many people fear the dark, so they choose to sleep with nightlights on or to fall asleep with the TV on. In addition, bedrooms can often become the catch-all for an overabundance of stuff that we do not want to leave out in the public areas of our homes. Whether books, magazines, papers, or clothes, the more our bedrooms become filled and busy, the poorer the air quality becomes.

Patterns of late night activity, or lack of it, also are powerful contributors to sleep disturbances. Though many are in denial about this, watching media where intense human drama, violence, and action are blasted out in rapid-fire images can be dizzying, affecting us energetically and emotionally. Pushing our bodies into the sympathetic nervous system—when we should be gearing down within the parasympathetic system of slowed respirations, heart rate activity, and digestion—prevents the relaxed state necessary for quality sleep. Swing shifts, night shifts, long shifts, and deadlines of all kinds are prescriptions for sleep difficulties.

"Fatigue is the best pillow."

—Benjamin Franklin

As children, we have resilience to these kinds of energy depletions, so during childhood, sleep deprivation seems not to affect us. As we continue to deplete energy through unhealthy practices, the deficiencies become increasingly apparent. That being said, it is also true that an increasing number of children are experiencing more problems sleeping. Their resilience may be being negatively affected even earlier by the combination of poor eating habits, living in a stressed family, having expectations for their performance that are too demanding, not having sufficiently healthy social interactions, and being too sedentary.

Adults are sleep deprived by as much as 1 to 1 1/2 hours per night. As a healthcare professional, I am much more aware of some of the horrific effects of prolonged sleep deprivation, but I find that my colleagues and I frequently fall into the same trap. Sleep deprivation affects judgment, memory, concentration, emotions, speech, and thought processes, and it often affects hormonal changes that increase weight gain.

"Sleeping is no mean art: for its sake one must stay awake all day."

—Friedrich Nietzsche

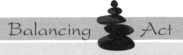

Balancing Act

## CATCHING YOUR ZZZZ'S

Ask yourself, "What are the behaviors and conditions in my life that might be reducing the quality of my sleep? In what ways have I been blinded by the choices I have made regarding my sleep?"

The following are some simple tips to help improve your sleep:

- If you're not ready to ban the TV, sound system, and other energy emitters from your bedroom, keep them on a power strip and completely unplug the power strip when you go to bed. This will minimize the energy output while you sleep.

- Don't eat within 2 hours of sleeping. Your organs need to be restoring themselves while you sleep, not trying to digest food.

- Don't drink caffeinated beverages past late afternoon.

- Declutter your bedroom to create a feeling of peace and harmony.

- Do deep breathing exercises before going to bed.

- When you're in bed, try to empty your mind. If you are concentrating on or worrying about falling asleep, you won't.

- Enjoy a warm cup of Lingzhi tea before bed.

For those who work in hospitals, there are additional challenges to getting sufficient sleep. Nurses are required to work double shifts if there is no staffing replacement, sometimes leaving at 1:00 a.m. and returning at 7:00 a.m. the next morning. We have become experts at prescribing and providing optimal care to our client population. Yet how many times over the years have we provided a similar standard of care for ourselves? How many of us felt that we could catch a 3-hour catnap before leaving for our next "tour of duty"? If we thought to pack a lunch, it is often consumed while driving or at the nurses' station or in the linen room. We dehydrate ourselves by not taking the time to drink sufficient water, but then dehydrate ourselves more by drinking coffee to stay awake. It is no wonder that when a working parent collapses into the sofa to spend time reading a favorite bedtime story to a child, the parent falls asleep before the story ends.

It is ironic that healthcare professionals are often compelled to work in systems that are strangely not designed to support our own health. Sleep deprivation then becomes a powerful contributor to professional burnout and compassion fatigue, both of which healthcare providers are at risk of developing.

When was the last time that you relived a favorite bedtime routine from your past? Do you remember the special feeling and aroma of a warm bath, clean pajamas, and freshly laundered sheets with a relaxing bedtime story and a cup of warm milk or bedtime tea? Do you remember "preparing" for bed?

*"A good laugh and a long sleep are the best cures in the doctor's book."*

—Irish Proverb

When was the most recent time that you awakened refreshed, full of energy, and ready to take on the challenges of a new day? Quality sleep is absolutely essential for physical and emotional well-being. Deep sleep without waking in the night (which decreases the amount of time spent in deep sleep and in the REM cycles) is necessary for body repair and restoration, immune system support, and coping with stress. The depth of the sleep, firmness and quality of the mattress, proper body alignment, and proper temperature are important variables in providing quality sleep.

Taking prescription or over-the-counter medications for sleep may facilitate the sleep cycle and sometimes can be lifesaving. But prescription medications are often prescribed without enough information about possible health risks, both in adjusting to the drug and in potential short- and long-term side effects. Too few doctors and patients know enough about alternatives to drugs to decrease or eliminate sleep challenges. And, over-the-counter products may present similar problems with side effects and interactions with other products. A natural approach related to mattress and pillow selection, linen choice, and eliminating distractors from the sleep area (power strips, cell phone chargers) is best.

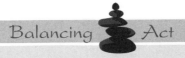

## MATTRESS MATTERS

Americans spend one-third of their lives sleeping, so it makes sense to invest in a sleep set that can improve your comfort and overall health. These tips are good to consider when selecting a mattress:

- **Shop for support:** Look for a mattress that provides uniform support from head to toe; if there are gaps between your body and the mattress (such as at the waist), you're not getting the full support you need. Mattresses can be too firm; pay close attention to uncomfortable pressure on prominent body features, such as the shoulders, hips, and low back. Because your body is pressing down on the springs at the low areas, these springs push back, creating pressure points. A pressure point can create the same effect as when you compress an injury to stop bleeding. That is, it restricts blood flow to these areas.

- **Shop for comfort:** When mattress shopping, give each option a good trial run before you buy; lie down on a mattress for a minimum of 5 to 10 minutes to get a good idea of its comfort level. If you cannot find a comfortable position, you probably have the wrong mattress.

- **Shop for size:** Does the bed provide enough room for you—and your sleeping partner if you have one—to stretch and roll over? The ideal mattress also minimizes the transfer of movement from one sleeping partner to the other, which means one person shouldn't feel motion as the other enters or leaves the bed.

The American Chiropractic Association (2007) is the source for the above information; they state that sleeping on a new mattress can significantly reduce stress as well as back pain.

Additionally, there are a number of specialized products you can consider:

- **Eco-functional bedding:** Eco-functional bedding is infused with properties that affect the sleep process. By infusing the functional materials—including chitin, bamboo charcoal, far infrared technology, and negative ions—within the fibers, the bedding retains its functions even after repeated machine washing and drying.

*continues*

continued

- **Organic mattress:** Many modern mattresses contain toxic chemicals used in the construction process that outgas and can harm your health and impede sleep. Organic mattresses use only organic materials without harmful chemicals.

- **Far-infrared technology:** Far-infrared energy is part of all living things. It is constantly absorbing energy and reflecting it as gentle warmth. Far-infrared absorbs moisture, reflects heat, and insulates the body. The technology offers all-season comfort.

- **Rubberthane technology:** A natural way to relieve stress and discomfort is with massage. Several sleep products attempt to reproduce this sensation with a textured or raised egg-carton-like surface similar to the egg-crate mattresses that we have used for years in healthcare. Every time that you move during sleep, the Rubberthane nodules help to ease tension and relax the body.

*"The best vitamin to be a happy person is B1."*

—Author Unknown

Sleep may be a challenge, especially for those working multiple shifts and irregular hours. Alternatives to sleep medication may include homeopathic blends, flower essences, and essential oils, all of which relax the body and mind, creating a good internal environment for restful sleep. Taking calcium and magnesium before bed, melatonin (unless contraindicated due to certain types of depression), valerian root extracts or teas, and kava kava are all excellent ways to promote better sleep and thus better mental health. Also consider seeing a chiropractor or nurse practitioner who specializes in glandular/hormonal balancing. Hormonal and glandular health is important to overall emotional/mental health. Remember, it is during REM sleep that memory is restored and cellular health is enhanced.

Sleep is not an option; it is not an elective that we can choose to use. Don't be sleepless in Seattle, or anywhere!

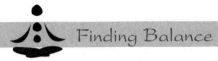

## REFLECTIONS

- Be aware of signs of sleep deprivation and take action
- Recharge your batteries
- Rest well, be well, and do well

# REFERENCES

Albuquerque, R. G., Hachul, H., Andersen, M. L., & Tufik, S. (2014). The importance of quality of sleep in menopause. *Climacteric*. doi:10.3109/136971 37.2014.888713

Allnurses. (2013). Lawsuit claims nurse was 'worked to death.' Retrieved from http://allnurses.com/general-nursing-discussion/lawsuit-claims-nurse-888155.html

Alphay. (n.d.). Eco-functional bedding. Retrieved from http://joinalphay.com

American Academy of Sleep Medicine. (2008). Circadian rhythm sleep disorders. Retrieved from http://www.aasmnet.org/resources/factsheets/crsd.pdf

American Chiropractic Association. (2007). Proper mattress can improve sleep comfort, reduce pain, says American Chiropractic Association. Retrieved from http://www.acatoday.org/press_css.cfm?CID=2541

Centers for Disease Control and Prevention (CDC). (n.d.). Insufficient sleep is a public health epidemic. Retrieved from http://www.cdc.gov/features/dssleep/

Cherry, K. (n.d.). Stages of sleep: The four stages of sleep. About.com Psychology. http://psychology.about.com/od/statesofconsciousness/a/SleepStages.htm

Chopra, D. (n.d.). How to get restful sleep. Retrieved from http://www.chopra.com/community/online-library/tips/how-to-get-restful-sleep

Morgenthaler, T. (2013). How many hours of sleep are enough for good health. The Mayo Clinic. Retrieved from http://www.mayoclinic.org/healthy-living/adult-health/expert-answers/how-many-hours-of-sleep-are-enough/faq-20057898

Mullington, J. M., Haack, M., Toth, M., Serrador, J. M., & Meier-Ewert, H. K. (2009). Cardiovascular, inflammatory, and metabolic consequences of sleep deprivation. *Progress in Cardiovascular Diseases, 51*(4), 294-302.

National Institute of General Medical Sciences. (n.d.). Circadian rhythm fact sheet. Retrieved from http://www.nigms.nih.gov/Education/Pages/Factsheet_CircadianRhythms.aspx

National Institute of Neurological Disorders and Stroke. (n.d.). Brain basics: Understanding sleep. Retrieved from http://www.ninds.nih.gov/disorders/brain_basics/understanding_sleep.html

Shaver, J. L., & Zenk, S. N. (2000). Review: Sleep disturbance in menopause. *Journal of Women's Health & Gender-Based Medicine, 9*(2), 109-118.

U.S. Department of Transportation (USDOT). (n.d.). *Drowsy driving and automobile crashes.* National Highway Traffic Safety Administration, National Center on Sleep Disorders Research. Retrieved from www.nhtsa.gov/people/injury/drowsy_driving1/Drowsy.html#NCSDR/NHTSA

*"Pull up a chair. Take a taste. Come join us. Life is so endlessly delicious."*

–Ruth Reichl

# 10

# BE HAPPY, EAT WELL, GET MOVING, LIVE LONGER, AND LIVE WELL

*–Sharon M. Weinstein, MS, RN, CRNI, FACW, FAAN*

"Waitress wanted. Must be able to swim underwater." That was the humorous sign posted in the window of a restaurant submerged in water during the Midwest floods several years ago. And, after a major earthquake hit San Francisco, one man put a sign on his damaged house that said, "House for rent. Some assembly required."

Humor is a constant reminder that life must, and does, go on. In spite of our overwhelming loss, deep down we know that laughter provides relief. We know that it helps us cope. We know, too, that if we can laugh, we will somehow get through it. Humor, no matter when it comes, helps us bear the unbearable.

You know you're getting old when you stoop to tie your shoes and wonder what else you can do while you're down there. What's so funny about getting old? Aging is an issue that creates dissonance in most of us. Rare is the card for a birthday over age 39 that talks about aging as a joyful, happy experience. My grandson had a theory that forty is a really big number, and no one has to be forty. Instead, you can be 39+1, 39+2, 39+3, and more. What a novel approach to the aging process; the idea itself brings me joy!

Knowing how to add humor to our conversations and to our activities keeps us happy, confident, and connected with others. Conflicts and differences of opinions are prevented or managed. Humorous comments help us see a situation realistically.

Laughing reduces the level of stress hormones and triggers the release of health-enhancing hormones like endorphins, which are the body's natural painkillers. Have something in your workplace that makes you happy, that fulfills you, and that makes you smile. Berk, Felten, Tan, Bittman, and Westengard also suggests that the body's response to repetitive laughter is similar to the effect of repetitive exercise (2001). Make wise choices—you are what you digest and you can eat your way to good health. These two factors alone will help you in your quest to live longer and to live well.

Despite the medical, lifestyle, and nutritional advances that contribute to greater health and the possibility of longer and healthier lives, we appear to be becoming less healthy. It has been suggested that in the United States this generation of children will be the first in generations to not live as long as their parents, mainly due to lifestyle choices. Yet, according to research at the University of Massachusetts Medical School (UMMS), the average American born today can expect to live nearly 4 years longer than a person born two decades ago. The study, published in the *American Journal of Public Health* (Stewart, Cutler, & Rosen, 2013) addressed measurement of the quality-adjusted life expectancy (QALE), which tells us much more than how long a person can expect to live. It reveals the relative quality of those added years in terms of physical, emotional, and mental well-being.

Our concepts of what it means to get old have everything to do with choices we make now about our health. Healthy lifestyle elements include nutrition, sleep, movement, and social support.

The choices we make impact our mood. Being merry is not easy to pull off for most of us who experience stress. Stress comes in many forms, including periodic stressful situations and deadlines; prolonged, seemingly intractable, stressful dynamics; health problems; and stress reactions from earlier and unhealed traumas in our lives. And with each of these kinds of stress, the level of stress experienced can run the full range from minimal to catastrophic stress. Stress is a key risk factor in all disease conditions affecting the delicate balance of body, mind, and spirit. What can we do? We can be merry, eat well, live longer, and live well! That's the focus of this chapter.

# BE MERRY

For those of us who devote our professional lives to helping others who are sick, suffering, and struggling, there are certain caveats and pitfalls in addition to the general issue of professionals overextending themselves. There are stressors in every work environment, and sometimes they make the situation unbearable and joyless. So, how does one "be merry" and celebrate the joy in life?

"I love people who make me laugh. I honestly think it's the thing I like most, to laugh. It cures a multitude of ills. It's probably the most important thing in a person."

—Audrey Hepburn

A state of vibrant health is our birthright. At our core level, we are vibrant, alive, positive, and happy. But sadly, life's experiences and the stress of daily existence cause our bodies to degenerate, our emotions to go absent without leave (AWOL), and our souls to feel disconnected.

"There is a thin line that separates laughter and pain, comedy and tragedy, humor and hurt."

—Erma Bombeck

When you are feeling more energy, it is much easier to make whatever changes you want to make. With more vitality, you participate more fully in other aspects of your life, are more able to attend to projects that have been building up, and begin to feel immediately better about yourself for accomplishing more and feeling more on top of your own life.

Emotional energy is the most important and vital energy we have. Kirshenbaum (2004) describes emotional energy as a personal energy crisis, or an epidemic. "Emotional energy is the precondition for everything we care about," Kirshenbaum says. "Everything worth doing that's difficult gets lost without it. Marriages fail when we run out of the emotional energy to reach one more time across the divide of anger and silence. Dreams die when we lack the emotional energy to hang in there in the face of all the obstacles" (Gottlieb, 2003). Having sufficient emotional energy is the result of learning to harmonize the needs, involvements, and choices that we make while sustaining sufficiently healthy lifestyles so that our bodies can generate the physical energy necessary to feel good. Emotional energy is renewable energy; it is the barometer of being balanced and healthy enough for living with vitality, enthusiasm, connection, fulfillment, and inner peace.

Without emotional energy, the stresses of daily life take a greater toll; with it, a number of things happen energetically that have profound effects on satisfaction and sense of fulfillment in the world. Other people are drawn to us when we have sufficient emotional energy, more opportunities seem to present themselves, and our interactions are more positive, which generates energy rather than absorbing it through negative dynamics and experiences.

"Nothing brings me more happiness than trying to help the most vulnerable people in society. It is a goal and an essential part of my life—a kind of destiny. Whoever is in distress can call on me. I will come running wherever they are."

—Princess Diana

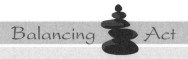

Balancing Act

# RECHARGE YOUR BATTERIES

The following suggestions can help you increase your energy, especially useful for those who are depressed and whose energy is depleted.

- Take 1 to 4 tablespoons of organic coconut oil daily. It goes right to the liver, rather than being dispersed through the lymphatic system, so it increases energy very quickly.

- Drink organic apple cider vinegar (2 teaspoons daily).

- Feel free to yawn; it cools down the brain.

- Use a deep-sleep mask with a washable cover that is far-infrared and infused with chitosan and bamboo charcoal. (You'll experience deep sleep within minutes.)

- Go to bed earlier. Even one hour earlier at night can make a noticeable difference the next morning. You may awaken feeling more refreshed and ready for the day. If you are already getting sufficient rest, the earlier sleep will provide extra energy and, because you'll probably awaken earlier, an early session of yoga, meditation, or prayer becomes more possible.

- Upon awakening, jot down all the early morning thoughts you have that you don't want to forget and then grab the mat for yoga or stretching to get the lymphatic system moving, stretch the muscles, and increase physical flexibility. This provides emotional and mental flexibility.

- Journal each morning and each night.

# LAUGHTER—THE BEST MEDICINE

Without question, one of the best feelings in the world is being overcome with uncontrollable laughter. You know the kind—when you laugh so hard you cry, and you keep chuckling each time you relive the moment, even hours after the "fit of laughter" has left you. According to Helpguide. org (2014), laughing, it turns out, has multiple health benefits:

*Physical*

- Boosts immunity
- Lowers stress hormones
- Decreases discomfort
- Prevents heart disease

*Mental*

- Adds joy to life
- Eases anxiety
- Is adaptogenic
- Improves resilience

*Social/Emotional*

- Strengthens relationships
- Improves teamwork
- Defuses tension
- Releases inhibitions

How does laughter do all of these things? Laughter affects these changes by raising the levels of infection-fighting proteins and cells that produce disease-destroying antibodies—T-cells and antibodies IgA and IgB. The thymus is responsible for distinguishing healthy cells from outside invaders. Joy, laughter, and happiness keep the thymus healthy. Laughter also helps with premenstrual syndrome (PMS) in a woman's menstrual cycle. And, laughter raises dehydroepiandrosterone (DHEA) levels; high levels of DHEA are a marker of health.

We live in a place and time in which very few things generate laughter, yet so much contributes to sadness and despair. Laughter is free of charge and readily available in multiple forms, including laughter yoga. Laughter yoga is a joyful and healthy exercise program using simulated laughter and breathing exercises taken from yoga. It is simple, and you do not need a reason to laugh! Developed by Dr. Madan Kataria, a physician from India, laughter yoga has spread across 72 countries and is easily done (Laughter Yoga International, 2014).

### Action Item

## LAUGHTER YOGA

- Laugh with guided techniques; you do not need a reason to laugh, yet laughter yields immediate benefits.

- Laughter is contagious; when we laugh as a group exercise, our childlike inner voice allows us to relax.

- Deep breathing associated with laughter yoga oxygenates the body and the brain; it is aerobic.

- Laughter generates positive energy.

- Laughter releases endorphins from the brain cells and enhances mood.

# HUMOR THROUGHOUT HISTORY

The American Holistic Nurses Association, in its *Core Curriculum for Holistic Nursing* (Dossey & Keegan, 2013), addresses the physiologic benefits of humor and laughter and calls laughter a wonderful tonic for the body. The core principles include:

- Humor as a cognitive skill that uses both sides of the brain

- Laughter as an antidote to stress

- Laughter increasing the number of helper T cells (Berk et al., 2001)

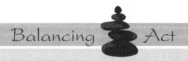

Balancing Act

# HUMOR THROUGHOUT HISTORY

**Biblical Times**

Book of Proverbs 17:22: "A cheerful heart does good like a medicine, but a broken spirit makes one sick."

**14th Century**

French surgeon Henri de Mondeville used humor therapy to enhance surgical recovery.

**16th Century**

Robert Burton, an English parson and scholar, used humor to cure melancholy.

Martin Luther used humor therapy for pastoral counseling.

**17th Century**

Herbert Spencer, sociologist, used humor to relieve tension.

**18th Century**

Immanuel Kant used humor to restore equilibrium.

William Battle used humor to treat the sick.

**20th Century**

Clowns were brought into U.S. hospitals to cheer children afflicted with polio.

The Gesundheit Institute was founded by Patch Adams (1972).

Norman Cousins published his book *Anatomy of an Illness as Perceived by the Patient* (1979) based on his own experiences using humor to recover from ankylosing spondylitis.

Release of *Patch Adams* film starring Robin Williams (1998).

**21st Century**

Laugh out loud (lol) therapy becomes a part of our daily lives through text messaging, emailing, instant messaging, and other forms of electronic communication.

Adapted from Laughter Therapy (http://www.freewebs.com/laughtertherapy/humourtherapy.htm).

World Laughter Day (1998) is celebrated annually the first Sunday in May. Traditionally laughter clubs across the world meet at midday to send a continual ripple of laughter around the world and to celebrate world peace through laughter.

# Psychology and Sociology of Laughter

Laughter is a universal, non-language-specific human phenomenon. The primary reason for laughter appears to be to bring people together (Provine, 2000). Bachorowski and Owren posit that we use laughter to elicit positive reactions from other people and to communicate to them that we mean them no harm (2003).

The range of laughter-arousing experiences is enormous, from physical tickling to mental titillations. Regardless of the cause of the laugher, it is an intellectual and emotional process enabling us to relieve pent-up emotions.

## Psychology and Society of Laughter

For years, our children referred to me as 50%, meaning that 50% of the time (or less), I had a good sense of humor. I actually "got" a joke; I could laugh at myself. I think that I have now graduated to 80%. Sometimes, I am the first to see the humor in a situation or to come up with a great line. Of course, family members are still amazed! Sometimes, I get "it"— whatever "it" might be! My level of awareness has increased as I have transitioned within my career from a focus on intervention to one of health and wellness (prevention and health promotion).

Laughter definitely has a place within every aspect of our lives. Laughter has enabled me to change my mind-set and shift my paradigms, and it has enhanced my well-being. As a professional, I have learned that we all need to assume responsibility for the joys of life! Let's face it; we sometimes work in stressful environments. Humor enables us to deal with stress more effectively; humor affects healing and recovery time; and, humor has enabled me to grow personally and professionally.

## HEALTH BENEFITS

What would we do without humor? How would we enjoy talks with others if we did not use humor to invite a smile or a laugh? And how would we manage the times when we feel sad and alone?

Humor lightens up each day and enables us to find common ground with others. We build healthy relationships with others by knowing what to say and do and also by knowing what hinders a conversation. Humor often takes us to the edge of uncertainty when we exaggerate or tease others to make our point. When humor is successful, we build trust and cooperation. We discover that we are not alone, we learn to accept our mistakes, and we look for the good in others and in ourselves. Essentially, we create common ground.

However, when we lose our senses of humor, we often get critical or defensive, and we blame others or ourselves for what has been said and the way in which it was said. Humor is an essential skill needed to communicate well with others. A few well-chosen words get the attention of others and make a serious point without creating a sense of defensiveness. Whether we prefer to be the center of attention or shy and quiet, humor can be adjusted to suit our personalities.

The challenge for everyone is to become more aware of how to add humor and when to avoid it. Too much humor, like too much spice, may annoy others. Humor that is perceived as insensitive may lead others to shut down or become argumentative. However, when we each maintain our sense of humor, we look for the good in others and in ourselves. To ensure that our humor is welcomed by others, we need to combine our humor with speaking clearly and listening effectively. That is clearly why we have two ears and a single mouth.

Much of our humor comes from reconnecting to our playful inner child. For many of us, it only takes a playful tone of voice, wearing a funny hat, or holding a stuffed toy to get started. Take a risk. Add a bit more humor to your day, and do it in a way that is right for you. When you are happy, you are light-hearted. You are open to others and ready to laugh and play.

## SMILE AND THE WORLD SMILES WITH YOU

As I have transitioned within my career, my sense of humor has definitely been a help. In my work with foreign ministers of health, education, and finance, I always needed to see the big picture of what was possible, but sometimes those things have not been probable. In my consulting practice, I have integrated humor in my work related to positive practice environments and wellness.

*"A smile starts on the lips, A grin spreads to the eyes, A chuckle comes from the belly; But a good laugh bursts forth from the soul, Overflows, and bubbles all around."*

*—Carolyn Birmingham*

## WATCH AND LAUGH

Here are some fun things to say to manage a stressful situation:

- You are terrific.
- Is it my turn to win?
- Is it too late to apologize?
- You're younger; you know best.
- My mother wants me to stop now.
- My father said...

Here are some fun things to do:

- Dance naked in front of your pets.
- Get a temporary tattoo.

- Eat dessert first.
- Make a handmade birthday card.
- Pop popcorn with the lid off.
- Tell stories about great personal successes or embarrassments.

Humor is the shortest distance between two people.

## THE CEDARS

At the 2007 Annual Meeting of the American Psychiatric Association in San Diego, California, researchers from Cedars-Sinai Medical Center showcased a study on brain tumors and laughter. The researchers investigated the dispositions toward humor of a group of depressed patients in the outpatient psychiatric department at Cedars-Sinai. Patients were asked to complete a short questionnaire comprised of a regular depression scale, as well as Svebak's Sense of Humor Questionnaire (Bokarius et al., 2011).

Svebak (2010), a professor at the Norwegian University of Science and Technology (NTNU), has examined the relationship between humor and health for years. He concludes that when you identify children as having a sense of humor, you may unintentionally include children who live an easy life. These children may not be quite as used to deal with later hardship as the less fortunate children. Children must be challenged, not unduly so, but enough to teach them how to react later in life, says Svebak.

In the Sinai presentation, Bokarius and colleagues (2011) shared the following benefits from laughter:

- Reduces cortisol levels in the body
- Improves circulation
- Stimulates nervous system
- Improves immune functioning
- Strengthens the heart
- Lowers blood pressure
- Releases endorphins

## PATCH ADAMS: A PIONEER

Perhaps Patch Adams was right all along about clowning around! I had the privilege of meeting the real Patch Adams at the International Council of Nurses (ICN) meeting several years ago. A gentleman and a scholar with an incredible sense of humor, Dr. Adams truly exemplified the philosophy that laughter is the best medicine.

In his book *Gesundheit* (Adams & Mylander, 1998), Patch Adams discusses his Vision for Building a Free Hospital and alludes to his medical school experience. He has also stated, "I entered medical school in 1967 to use medicine as a vehicle for social change" (Adams, n.d., para. 1). He could not conceive of a community that did not care for its people. Compassion and attention are a cry for time, and time is what was given by caregivers to patients. He continued, "The idea that a person was healthy because of normal lab values and clear x-rays had no relationship to who the person was. Good health was much more deeply related to close friendships, meaningful work, a lived spirituality of any kind, an opportunity for loving service and an engaging relationship to nature, the arts, wonder, curiosity, passion and hope. All of these are time-consuming, impractical needs. When we don't meet these needs, the business of high-tech medicine diagnoses mental illness and treats with pills" (Salt, 2012).

Therefore, activity within the hospital was infused with fun, and Adams created the first silly hospital in history. The silly hospital sought an ideal staff: those people who were naturally happy, fun loving, cooperative, and creative. There were no salaries and staff often worked part-time jobs in order to sustain themselves and their families. Without funding, the silly hospital faced overwhelming challenges. Adams then went public to secure funding to sustain the facility and to build a modern physical plant. Although the land was secured and a school of social change evolved, the actual hospital remained a dream. However, the model remains one of social change and healing arts. Patch Adams's example of joyful persistence is an important, inspiring model for the changes needed in the world.

Clown healing is now a regular part of hospitals on every continent, and the practice is expanding as people hear the message that it is really about spreading joy in every public space as gestures toward peace, justice, and care prevail. The message of laughter as the best medicine has spread worldwide, and the result is a newfound interest in Patch Adams's work. Laughter is indeed a powerful medicine—the best medicine! Laughter can fight disease by strengthening the immune system, protecting us against anything from the common cold to cancer. With today's hectic pace, we may need a few moments of laughter. It is free of charge and readily available.

## Learning to Laugh

You can, and should, learn to laugh. Those who love fun have their own ways of creating humor.

Here is what fun-loving people do away from work:

- Put up streamers even when there is no special occasion
- Make a family photo collage for the wall
- Make a hanging mobile for the house
- Wear funny hats in public
- Make music out of utensils from the kitchen

Don't forget humor in your personal life, too. Remember, a smile goes a long way, and laughter will:

- Promote a positive environment
- Create a sense of trust
- Cheer you and others around you
- Release tension
- Reduce stress
- Work the diaphragm

## Work Setting

Here is what businesses have done to improve communication with employees and keep a sense of balance across the organization:

- Wheeling around a refreshment cart at 3:00 p.m. on Fridays
- Replacing dress down Fridays with dress up Fridays

- Celebrating birthdays each month with a cake and a get-together at lunch

In office-work environments, you can

- Decorate your office with toys that you and your visitors can play with when things get difficult. Play dough is a great office tool!
- Make those around you laugh at least three times a day and they will return the favor.
- Keep silly photos of you and your loved ones around you.
- Keep "dress up" items like silly costumes found at garage or yard sales in your office.

## PATIENT CARE

Laughter has enormous health benefits for those with a diversity of clinical situations, from helping those with chronic diseases, such as diabetes, to lowering risk of heart attacks and everything in between. In the world in which we live, which is replete with modern medical breakthroughs, who would ever dream that something as simple as laughter could induce such amazing benefits for your health?

## LOVE LIFE

Remember: Laughter is contagious. Have something in your workplace that automatically makes you smile (Scott, 2011). After you're smiling, spread it around and make your coworkers smile, too! You've learned how to laugh; now, it's time to look at how, and what, we ingest.

# EAT WELL

To examine your own blinders regarding eating and foods, take a mental walk through your local grocery store or supermarket. How much of what you find is fresh? How much is natural? How much is organic? It shouldn't take an outbreak of E-coli in spinach or salmonella in tomatoes to convince you it's in your best interest to know how your food is grown, what is used to grow it, and where it comes from. Remember to retain your habits, but to change your choices!

*"Remember me with smiles and laughter, for that is how I will remember you all. If you can only remember me with tears, then don't remember me at all"*
*—Laura Ingalls Wilder*

The focus of this book is on recommending that you know what you are eating. The Internet, the news, celebrity experts like Dr. Oz, and the media have told us repeatedly that diet and health are intimately connected.

## You Are What You Digest

Although you might be familiar with the phrase, "You are what you eat," you might not know that you are what you digest. Digestion plays a major role in health.

## Eating In and Out

Can you remember when the family meal was a time where all family members were together engaging in a ritual that brought cohesion, relaxation, good conversation, and laughter, which are all great elements for proper digestion? Perhaps your family runs from the school to the practice field, from enrichment activities to meetings, and dinner as a family happens only on the weekend. It is not too late to create your own rituals, traditions, and lasting memories now, even if it requires adjustments in routines that have become commonplace.

As overextended professionals, we are more likely to eat to try to increase our energy. At these times, we typically choose foods that spike our insulin levels. They also tend to be ones that are easiest to get into our mouths quickly and on the go. The easiest are too often the worst for us: highly refined, processed, and packaged foods. Most restaurants will cater to special dietary requests and have gluten-free or other alternatives. Never hesitate to ask for healthful choices. And, if you choose to eat organically, ask chefs about the sources of their food. They are more likely to source from local and sustainable sources if customers ask.

## Balancing Act

## GOOD, GOOD, GOOD, GOOD DIGESTION

1. **Chew until liquid.** By chewing foods until they've liquefied, two things are accomplished: First, tremendous burden is taken off of the stomach and intestines, allowing for more energy to be available for healing, repair, and maintenance of tissues and organs. Secondly, chewing foods until they've liquefied enables powerful digestive enzymes in saliva to thoroughly mix with food, which is an essential first step for optimal digestion.

2. **Minimize drinking water and other fluids while eating.** Drinking water and other fluids can cause dilution of stomach acids and digestive enzymes, making them less effective at breaking down food. Whenever possible, it is best to drink fluids before and 2 hours after meals.

3. **Avoid physical exertion following meals.** Approximately one-half of the body's entire blood supply is needed by the digestive organs following a meal. Physical exertion diverts blood away from our digestive organs, thereby reducing the efficiency of the digestive processes. Taking time to physically rest for approximately 1 hour following meals will allow for adequate blood supply to the digestive organs and optimal digestion.

*Source: http://drbenkim.com/*

## NUTRIENTS

Even if you eat only the best foods, follow optimal digestion practices, exercise, and take care of yourself in other ways, you may still need nutrient supplementation to achieve increased energy and health. An acidic body is an unhealthy body. Make an effort to eat a balanced diet and to drink a sufficient amount of water. The more you eat according to the specific needs of your body, the healthier you will continue to be and the younger you will look and feel. Consider consulting with a nutritionist, nurse practitioner, or holistic professional to ascertain your nutrient, pH, hormone, and enzyme levels to determine the best supplementation for you. Remember: all supplements are not created equal.

# HEALTHY LIVING 101

Remember that healthy living does not begin in the physician's office; it begins with the small decisions that we make each day when we pack our kids' lunches, shop for groceries, or order from a menu. We can, and should, control our health!

# EATING FOR THE SEASON

Consider the benefits of eating foods at their peak season. Seasonal foods serve up the most flavor, pack the biggest nutritional punch, and can also boost your budget.

# HEALTHY SHOPPING

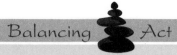

Balancing Act

## TIPS FOR BUYING PRODUCE

1. In *spring,* buy apricots, artichokes, asparagus, avocados, beets, carrots, cauliflower, cherries, English peas, radishes, and spinach. A few tips: Avocados should be slightly soft and squeezable. Apricots should have a uniform color and shape and be slightly soft, as well. Spinach should have bright green, crisp leaves.

2. In *summer,* buy berries, corn, cucumbers, eggplant, figs, and garlic. Berries usually have a nice aroma when they're ripe.

3. In *fall,* buy apples, arugula, broccoli, fennel, hard-shelled squash, pears, persimmons, pomegranate, sweet peppers, and sweet potatoes. Squash shouldn't have soft spots.

4. In *winter*, broccoli rabe is the most well-known piece of produce.

*Source: eHow.com*

## PURCHASE ORGANICALLY OR CHEMICAL-FREE

The following produce is highest in pesticide residue. It's good to buy organic varieties of these fruits and vegetables:

| | |
|---|---|
| Peaches | Berries |
| Apples | Lettuce |
| Sweet Bell Peppers | Pears |
| Celery | Spinach |
| Nectarines | |

The following fruits and vegetables are the lowest in pesticide residue:

| | |
|---|---|
| Onions | Bananas |
| Avocado | Cabbage |
| Pineapples | Broccoli |
| Asparagus | Eggplant |
| Kiwi | |

*Source: http://www.ewg.org/consumer-guides*

"Honestly, I just try to live right, get enough sleep, and drink a lot of water. I do drink a lot of water; I do live by that. And just eating good clean food…. I do love all of it. But I do definitely try to eat better organic food."

—Keshia Knight Pulliam

## DAIRY

Since 1993, a synthetic growth hormone, recombinant Bovine Growth Hormone (rBGH), has been injected into U.S. dairy cows to artificially increase milk production (Health Care Without Harm, n.d.). Both the American Nurses Association (ANA) (Health Care Without Harm, n.d.) and Physicians for Social Responsibility (2003) have issued policy statements against dairy products produced from cows injected with rBGH . Both organizations state specifically the increase in disease rates in rBGH-injected cows and the potential for harm to humans, the increase in antibiotic use in rBGH-injected cows which could lead to antibiotic resistance in humans, the potential cancer risk in humans through greater levels of insulin-like growth factor (IGF-1), and the fact that 30 countries to date have banned rBGH-injected dairy products.

## MEAT

Most meats sold in large-scale grocery and big-box stores—beef, pork, chicken, and turkey—are from animals raised on industrial/factory farms that are sometimes referred to as Concentrated Animal Feeding Operations (CAFOs). CAFOs are agricultural facilities that house and feed a large number of animals in a confined area for 45 days or more during any 12-month period. These are factory farms that practice raising farm animals in high-density populations to optimize profit. Confinement practices create situations that can be conducive to disease and lameness (Union of Concerned Scientists, 2008). Thus, most animals in CAFOs and other factory farms are prophylactically fed antibiotics to promote quick growth and to compensate for crowded, stressful, unsanitary conditions. Some CAFOs also supply tranquilizing drugs in the feed or water to keep the stressed animals calmer and to prevent potential injuries.

*"The way you cut your meat reflects the way you live."*
*—Confucius*

## CDC Statement

The Centers for Disease Control and Prevention (CDC) have a statement posted on their website addressing CAFOs:

## Public Health Concerns

People who work with livestock may develop adverse health effects, including chronic and acute respiratory illnesses and musculoskeletal injuries, and they may be exposed to infections that travel from animals to humans. Residents in areas surrounding CAFOs report nuisances, such as odor and flies. In studies of CAFOs, the CDC has shown that chemical and infectious compounds from swine and poultry waste are able to migrate into soil and water near CAFOs. Scientists do not yet know whether or how the migration of these compounds affects human health.

Pollutants possibly associated with manure-related discharges at CAFOs include:

- **Antibiotics**, which may contribute to the development of antibiotic-resistant pathogens

- **Pathogens**, such as parasites, bacteria, and viruses, which can cause disease in animals and humans

- **Nutrients**, such as ammonia, nitrogen, and phosphorus, which can reduce oxygen in surface waters, encourage the growth of harmful algal blooms, and contaminate drinking-water sources

- **Pesticides and hormones**, which researchers have associated with hormone-related changes in fish

- **Solids**, such as feed and feathers, which can limit the growth of desirable aquatic plants in surface waters and protect disease-causing microorganisms

- **Trace elements**, such as arsenic and copper, which can contaminate surface waters and possibly harm human health

*Source: http://www.vegansoapbox.com/*
*public-health-concerns-of-factory-farms/*

For many healthcare professionals, there is a significant concern that overuse of antibiotics in the food chain is contributing to antibiotic-resistant bacteria strains in animals and humans.

## CONSUMERISM

Be an educated consumer, even when it comes to the layout of the supermarket. Today, we see more people than ever before purchasing groceries online. Whether onsite or online, it is essential to have a list, know how to read and interpret labels, and raise your own awareness of food labelling. Don't shop on an empty stomach; you may end up buying things that you do not need, but that you are eager to taste during the shopping experience.

## ALPHABET SOUP

Shopping has become an alphabet experience! The following sections describe what those acronyms and words really mean.

### GMO

Genetically modified organisms (GMOs) are plants or animals whose cells have been modified to specific characteristics. For example, plants might be genetically engineered to develop a resistance against insects or to increase nutrients. There are both health and environmental concerns about GMOs. The most common genetically modified foods are corn, canola, soybean, and cotton. No genetically engineered animals have been approved for sale for human consumption in the United States.

### Proposition 65

The State of California has Proposition 65 (http://oehha.ca.gov/prop65/prop65_list/newlist.html), which is often referred to as the heavy metals standard. Its purpose is to notify consumers that they are being exposed to chemicals that are known to cause cancer and/or reproductive toxicity. A Proposition 65 warning does not necessarily mean a product is in violation of any product-safety standards or requirements.

## Vegan

Veganism is the practice of abstaining from animal products; it is more of a lifestyle choice than a diet. Vegans enjoy pizza, casseroles, burritos, chocolate cake, soups, and the other lifestyle foods that we all enjoy; they just do so without the use of animal products. Those who "go vegan" do so for health, environmental, and ethical reasons.

## Gluten-Free

A gluten-free diet excludes foods containing gluten. A gluten-free diet is the only medically accepted treatment for celiac disease, yet people from all walks of life are proclaiming themselves gluten-free. This may be because of digestive issues or gluten sensitivity, which leads to stomach cramps, diarrhea, and bloating. Unfortunately, some people also refer to this diet plan as the secret to quick weight loss. Of course, one loses weight simply because there are fewer food choices available, and consequently consumption decreases.

## Organic

Shopping organic is about safety and the environment. Organic dairy farmers and ranchers use pure water, quality feed, fresh air, and healthy pastures to make sure their organically raised animals grow at a natural pace and without artificial growth hormones. Current U.S. Department of Agriculture (USDA) regulations allow food products that contain 95 to 100% certified organic ingredients to use the USDA Organic seal (http:// www.ams.usda.gov/AMSv1.0/ams.fetchTemplateData.do?template=Temp lateN&navID=NOSBlinkNOSBCommittees&rightNav1=NOSBlinkNO SBCommittees&topNav=&leftNav=&page=NOPOrganicStandards&res ultType=&acct=nopgeninfo).

## Kosher

Kosher foods are those prepared in accordance with Jewish dietary laws. Pork, rabbit, owl, catfish, sturgeon, and any shellfish are not kosher. Other types of meat and fowl must be slaughtered in a prescribed manner to be considered kosher. Newer standards include foods that are eco-kosher, meaning that they comply with Jewish dietary laws as well as consider industrial agriculture, global warming, and fair treatment of workers. Definitions have varied over time, and today's consumers for kosher foods include those people of other faiths who share concerns for food handling and preparation.

## Halal

Halal foods are those that are allowed under Islamic dietary guidelines. This excludes pork or pork by-products, animals that were dead prior to slaughtering, and blood and blood by-products.

## Convenience and Processed Foods

Most of us today were raised with convenience foods. It has become our habit to rely on convenient, processed, prepared food. Hectic work schedules lead to overuse of convenience and fast food. Eating while driving or working and during stressful business meals detracts from our balance and makes digestion difficult. Make a point of setting aside time to eat. Even if you cannot get away from fast food or fast casual right away, make time to eat at a table, not at your desk or in your car. It's a first step, but an important one. Set a goal for weaning yourself off fast food. For microwavable foods, read the labels. In general, regardless of how you prepare your meals, don't buy anything that has more than five ingredients or ingredients you cannot pronounce or you cannot identify.

*"Sugar is a type of bodily fuel, yes, but your body runs about as well on it as a car would."*

*—V. L. Allineare*

# IMPACT OF EXERCISE AND MOVEMENT

We know that if we consume less and move more, we might be able to control our weight. Many of us are challenged by working in jobs that require little movement. Do the following statements describe you?

- You sit at your desk for long periods of time.
- You have back/neck/shoulder pain.
- You have poor eating habits.

There are tips and techniques that you can implement to stay fit as you sit. The environment in which you work plays a key role in your overall well-being. You can take ownership of your mind and body and get to the very core of wellness.

Take a 15 to 20 minute walk instead of a coffee break. Walk at least 10,000 steps per day (use a pedometer). Sit up straight while you work and avoid slouching. Adjust your seat properly, and don't be afraid to stretch at your desk. Get out of your chair hourly. Do ankle rotations while you're seated. Skip the elevator and take the stairs. Lunge the stairs. Do abs at your desk by contracting six times slowly, quickly, slowly and the repeat the process. Squeeze your abs forcefully, sit upright and repeat. You can also work your arms by raising your elbows to shoulder level. Turn your torso slowly to the right as far as possible, and then to the left as far as you can go; repeat this 10 times. If you have a job that requires constant activity, perhaps in a clinical area, take adequate breaks.

*"The hardest thing about exercise is to start doing it. Once you're doing it, the hardest thing is to stop it."*

*—Erin Gray*

# Living Longer and Living Well

We all want to live longer, but we also want to live well, don't we? How can we make that happen? What are the factors involved in this evolving process? On a visit to Nantong, China, I was told about a village in which there were 800 people more than 100 years of age, each of whom was well and none of whom took medication. I was intrigued. What could they have been doing that enabled them to be well and to stay well—to live longer and to live well? I certainly wanted some of what they had for myself and my own family. I discovered that their secret was medicinal mushrooms, specifically the Lingzhi/Ganoderma/Reishi mushroom, often known as the herb of longevity.

> *"According to the time-honored 5 Elements of Heath and Balance, the foundation of Chinese Medicine, each of the body's major organ systems are nourished by Lingzhi; thus, it is said to balance all 5 Elements of the body, mind and spirit. In many ways, Lingzhi, and the other edible mushrooms found in all Alphay products can be considered to be the 'vehicles' for transporting important nutritional constituents into the physical body.*
>
> *In ancient texts and records, it is written that China was the first country to study the miraculous medicinal and healing properties of the Lingzhi mushroom. Known as 'lucky grass,' it is revered as a symbol of luck and happiness, and the mythology of Lingzhi has been passed from generation to generation for thousands of years"* (Alphay International, Inc., 2014).

I, too, have been consuming Lingzhi and other medicinal mushrooms for nearly 3 years, and I have seen my own profound health improvements.

Let's explore the idea of living longer and living well and see how paradigms have shifted.

## SHIFTING PARADIGMS

Paradigms have shifted; our concept of what is old has changed dramatically. How long ago did you think that people who are 60 or 70 were old, and what is considered old today?

The Baby Boomers have literally transformed every phase of human life and they fear getting older. Aging is inevitable, but it can be more pleasant in the absence of disease and discomfort.

### Dementia

Dementia facilities seem to be appearing on the landscape nationwide. Dementia is not part of normal aging; it is simply multiple cognitive deficits with memory impairments as an early symptom.

### Memory

A key concern among aging populations is memory loss. We all have those moments when we misplace the car keys, forget to lock the door, or cannot locate the document we are seeking. There are variables in the term "memory loss." Occasional lapses in memory are normal in both aging adults and in the rest of the population.

Mild cognitive impairment (MCI) occurs more often in aging populations than in the average person, but it does not prevent them from carrying on daily activities. Finally, age-related memory impairment (AMI) or age-associated memory impairment (AAMI) involves the ability to encode new memories of events or facts.

### Cognition

So what is normal with respect to cognitive skills and aging? Crystalized intelligence, obtained over time, remains stable with age; this is good news. Fluid intelligence, the ability to respond and react quickly, tends to decline. Think about the last time that you saw a senior citizen behind the wheel of a car, and you wondered about his or her ability to respond and react quickly. It may take longer to get the words out, but the words are definitely there and processing takes a bit longer.

*"Memory is the fourth dimension to any landscape."*
—Janet Fitch

## Agility

Changes in agility have a significant effect on aging. I see people my own age who have become less agile as they've aged, but then I've also read about a 90-year-old yoga expert. The ability to climb stairs, run a mile, sit, and stand differs from one person to another. There are steps that we can take to enhance agility as we age; hydration is one of them. We found out long ago that Ponce de Leon's fountain of youth was probably a notion rather than truth. The consequences of lifestyle and disease impact one's agility.

## Balance

Balance issues are a frequent cause for concern as one ages. Fears of falling on the ice, getting fractures, and experiencing age-related dizziness and imbalance are all too real. Sometimes these problems evolve as a result of over-medicating those who are growing older. When systems slow down, the dose of medication should be adjusted to ensure proper distribution and absorption by the body. Balance problems may even be related to the inner ear, circulation, or vision. Occasionally imbalance is related to a heart disorder, or perhaps a nervous system disorder. An awareness of changes in balance is the first step toward resolution. The most common types of imbalance are vertigo, lightheadedness, and unsteadiness.

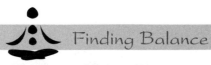

Finding Balance

## FINDING YOUR BALANCE

Take this simple self-awareness test and be merry, eat well, keep moving, live longer, and live well from this point forward.

On a scale from 0 to 10, where 10 represents the best possible it seems that one could feel (not necessarily you because you might have the tendency to downplay how good you could feel) how would you rate yourself with each of the following states:

- What is the worst you ever felt emotionally?
- What is the worst you ever felt physically/ energetically?
- What is the healthiest you ever felt?
- What is the happiest you ever felt?
- How good do you believe you can feel?
- How good (physically, emotionally, and energetically) are you feeling now?

Answering these questions gives you both a baseline and a road map for yourself as you continue to improve your overall state of well-being. Use these numbers to track your efforts and your experience daily. You could also use this to track how well you ate, how well you slept, how much energy you have, how bright your mood is. Tracking how often and what kind of exercise you do, what kind of centering/grounding you do (meditation, prayer, and so on), is an excellent way to increase your awareness of how much your lifestyle choices affect your well-being and how well you are really feeling.

## REFLECTIONS

So, laugh a little, eat well, move more, live longer, and live well by

- Taking care of *you*
- Taking the time to enjoy life and to smile
- Moving more and maintaining balance

# REFERENCES

Adams, P. (n.d). Vision for a free hospital based on fun and friendship. Gesundheit Institute. Retrieved from http://patchadams.org/hospital_project

Adams, P., & Mylander, M. (1998). *Gesundheit! Bringing good health to you, the medical system, and society through physician service, complementary.* San Francisco: Robert D. Reed.

Alphay International, Inc. (2014). Lingzhi Culture: A 2,000 year old tradition. Retrieved from http://www.alphayglobal.com/Company/Lingzhi

Bachorowski, J.-A., & Owren, M. J. (2003). Sounds of emotion: The production and perception of affect-related vocal acoustics. *Annals of the New York Academy of Sciences, 1000*, 244-265.

Berk, L. S., Felten, D. L., Tan, S. A., Bittman, B. B., & Westengard, J. (2001). Modulation of neuroimmune parameters during the eustress of humor-associated mirthful laughter. *Alternative Therapies in Health and Medicine, 7*(2): 62-72, 74-76.

Bokarius, A., Ha, K., Poland, R., Bokarius, V., Rapaport, M., and Ishak, W. (2011). Attitude toward humor in patients experiencing depressive symptoms. *Innovations in Clinical Neuroscience, 8*(9), 20-23.

Dossey, B. M., & Keegan, L. (2013). *Core curriculum for holistic nursing.* Boston, MA: Jones & Barlett.

Gottlieb, A. (2003). 8 energy zappers—and how to avoid them. *O Magazine.* Retrieved from http://www.oprah.com/omagazine/Solving-the-Emotional-Energy-Crisis

Health Care Without Harm. (2014). Nurses rBGH-Free Dairy Toolkit. Retrieved from https://noharm-uscanada.org/content/us-canada/nurses-rbgh-free-dairy-toolkit

Helpguide.org. (2014). Laughter is the best medicine. Retrieved from http://www.helpguide.org/life/humor_laughter_health.htm

Kirshenbaum, M. (2004). *The emotional energy factor.* New York, NY: Bantam.

Laughter Yoga International. (2014). Laughter yoga: Health and fitness craze sweeping the world. Retrieved from http://www.laughteryoga.org/english/laughteryoga/details/97

Physicians for Social Responsibility. (2003). Campaign for safe food. Retrieved from http://www.psr.org/chapters/oregon/safe-food/campaign-for-safe-food.html

Provine, R. (2000). The science of laughter. *Psychology Today.* Retrieved from http://www.psychologytoday.com/articles/200011/the-science-laughter

Salt, S. (2012). Laughter nothing to sneeze at. Cleveland.com. Retrieved from http://blog.cleveland.com/healing//print.html?entry=/2012/04/laughter_nothing_to_sneeze_at.html

Scott, B. (2011, February 22). Study: For a better workday, smile like you mean it. Retrieved from http://www.eurekalert.org/pub_releases/2011-02/msu-sfa022211.php

Stewart S. T., Cutler, D. M., & Rosen, A. B. (2013). US trends in quality-adjusted life expectancy from 1987 to 2008: Combining national surveys to more broadly track the health of the nation. *American Journal of Public Health, 103*(11), e78-87.

Svebak, S. (2010). The sense of humor questionnaire: Conceptualization and revision of 40 years of finding in empirical research. *Europe's Journal of Psychology, 6*(3). Retrieved http://ejop.psychopen.eu/article/view/218

Union of Concerned Scientists. (2008). CAFOs Uncovered: The untold costs of confined animal feeding operations. Retrieved from http://www.ucsusa.org/food_and_agriculture/our-failing-food-system/industrial-agriculture/cafos-uncovered.html

"That is the great fallacy: the wisdom of old men.
They do not grow wise, they grow careful."

—Ernest Hemingway

# 11

# REINVENTING YOURSELF: BECOMING MORE OF YOU

*—Sharon M. Weinstein, MS, RN, CRNI, FACW, FAAN*

Now that you've reflected on and made strides toward balancing all
aspects of your life, it's time to consider *who* that rebalanced you becomes in the workplace. Has your path led you to a forked road where
"straight ahead" is no longer an option? Perhaps this is a personal
choice or because the organization has changed and your skills no
longer fit the new business focus. Or, are you merely at a crossroads
where you can continue on your present course but want to consider
the options other directions offer? Regardless of what brought you to
your present place, it may be time to step back, take a deep breath, and
reflect on a new vision of what a career might mean for you.

# Going Forward or Stepping Back

Realizing you need change to get out of your rut is the first step. After you've made that realization, spend some time thinking about which direction you want to go. Do you want to change into a new career? Stay in the same career but move forward into a promotion? Stay in the same career but move backward into a prior job that you enjoyed, that was more meaningful, and that was less stressful? Segue into an "unjob" (contract, freelance, or self-employment work) or put your career on hold (sabbatical or leave of absence) while you explore those things you always wanted to do that offer zero or minimal financial compensation? This could mean honing an art like pottery or painting or even exploring missionary work. Take the time to reflect on how your life purpose and your dreams should direct your career choices. Many of the exercises throughout the chapters can also be applied to career exploration. See the "Career-Change Exercises" sidebar for some career-specific exercises. A good resource on the Web is Quintessential Careers (http://www.quintcareers.com/career-changer.html).

*"Everyone thinks of changing the world, but no one thinks of changing himself."*

—Leo Tolstoy

Balancing Act

# CAREER-CHANGE EXERCISES

Career change can occur for a number of reasons, from the anticipated (marriage, empty nest) to the unexpected (illness, divorce, layoff) to "non-events" (a promotion that fell through, a friend got promoted).

## Reflection: SWOT analysis

If you are looking for a career change to advance your own career then the SWOT (Strengths, Weaknesses, Opportunities, Threats) analysis is an excellent tool for getting an accurate and informed view of where you are right now. You should use it before making any decisions about future career choice.

The SWOT analysis shown in the example asks you to consider the following factors:

- What are your strengths?

- What are your weaknesses or development needs?

- What are the opportunities for development within your chosen career?

- What threats are you facing?

Use the following guide in thinking about the types of areas you should explore in your personal SWOT analysis. The analysis will help in clarifying career choices, such as whether to move into another role within your current organization or to exit the organization.

## Strengths

- What do you consider to be your most marketable skills?

- How can your skills transfer to other roles in your organization, other functional areas, and other industries?

- What are your best leadership qualities?

## Opportunities

- What is the level of demand for the skill sets that you possess in your organization or your preferred organization?

- What type of advertising is being planned?

- What development strategies could you adopt to increase your chances of landing a role?

| Weaknesses | Threats |
|---|---|
| • What gaps in capability do you perceive you have for the role you aspire to? | • Who in the organization will be a resistance or block to you moving into this role? |
| • What would others say are your blind spots? | • What is the level of competition for this role? |
| • How might your blind spots derail your potential? | • Have you resigned in difficult circumstances? How will you explain this in your next interview? |

You can effectively plan and manage career change through career choice analysis and the ways you choose to develop your career.

# WHEEL OF LIFE—GET THE BALANCE RIGHT

A week consists of 168 hours. Measure and reflect on the past 3 months and estimate the time you have spent on the following eight aspects of your life:

- **Business:** Career progression activity

- **Finance:** Investments and other monetary activities and responsibilities

- **Family:** Spouse, kids, parents, and other relatives

- **Spiritual:** Worship, Community, Volunteering

- **Physical:** General exercise, sports, or activity participation

- **Mental:** Reading, self-learning, formal education

- **Social:** Friends, outings, movies, having fun

- **Rest:** Sleep, "me time," relaxation, holidays

Generally if any one of these parts of your life is taking up a lot of your time over a sustained period, other areas of your life suffer. Your career should be your passion and contribute to your overall happiness and well-being.

*Source: Everybody's Career Company,*
*www.reinventyourcareer.com.au/*

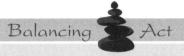

Balancing Act

## RETIRE OR REWIRE?

Ask yourself the following questions. Then, examine your responses and identify what you must do in order to be balanced. For example, if the items on your bucket list are out of reach, you need to change something in your schedule to allow you to have those experiences.

1. Identify the people, places, and activities that give you joy today.

2. What is your vision for your future?

3. List five things on your bucket list.

4. Do you plan to work beyond age 60?

5. Do you plan to always do the same kind of work?

6. What will change for you if you change careers?

7. What will change for you if you stop working?

8. Do you currently do volunteer work or serve on a board?

9 Are you and your life partner on the same page?

# STAYING IN OR STARTING A NEW JOB—LIVE A PASSIONATE LIFE

We want to feel passionate about the work that we do and define our contribution to mankind, our purpose for being. We want to know that we are contributing to the greater good and that our life has meaning. We want to find our calling, but do we know what that calling really is?

*"Don't ask yourself what the world needs; ask yourself what makes you come alive. And then go and do that. Because what the world needs is people who have come alive."*

—Harold Whitman

It would be so much easier if, during high school, we were sent a directive for our life's work. It would be so much easier if we went to university having already decided on a major and maintained that major through graduation. It would be so much easier if our class schedule remained a constant, if our first selection of an employer was the right one for us, and if our selection of a life's partner was also the right one from the start. However, life is not like that. We are not handed directives that will last throughout our lives. Instead, life is a process, and by going through the process we focus on an evolution of ourselves through time.

# PERSONALITY TYPES

Regardless of your career path, the process remains just that—a process. You can facilitate that process, in addition to the SWOT analysis, by knowing who you are. There are a number of psychometric tools that evaluate personality style, aptitude, and skill sets. Myers-Briggs Type Indicator (MBTI) is probably one of the better known tools (Cunningham, 2012). I took this assessment with a former employer. The results were amazing; I scored 25% in each of the four quadrants; only the president of the company and I had this outcome.

The purpose of the MBTI personal inventory is to understand type theory. The assessment looks at where you direct your energy (extraversion/introversion); how you process information (sensing/intuition); how you make decisions (thinking/feeling); and how you prefer to organize your life (judging/perception). When you decide on your preference in each category, your personality type is defined. There is no best type; it's just further evidence of the fact that we are all unique. In my workplace the MBTI was used to identify internal power partners with whom employees might best work and/or collaborate.

There are other types of personality tests available. A favorite of mine is the 5 Elements assessment (Chen, 2011), which is also tied to the seasons and even the systems within the human body.

| Element and Strength | Wood Leader | Fire Inspirer | Earth Diplomat | Metal Observer | Water Philosopher |
|---|---|---|---|---|---|
| Style | Decision-maker | Natural net-worker | Giver | Detail-oriented | Big dreamer |
| Needs | Acts | Excitement | Nurturing | Time to learn | Guidance |
| Desires | To motivate others | Fulfillment | Connectedness | Order | Integrity |
| Emotions | Helplessness | Isolation | Being lost | Corruption | Lack of visibility |
| Seeks | Causes | Appreciation | To defuse difficult settings | Systems | Learning |
| Weakness | Controller | Performer | Rescuer | Inflexible | Invisible |

For example, each of the five elements is related to the following internal systems:

Wood (Spring): liver and gallbladder, vision

Fire (Summer): heart, small intestine, pericardium

Earth (Indian Summer): spleen and stomach

Metal (Autumn): lungs and large intestine

Water (Winter): kidneys and bladder

Women and caregivers are often high in the Earth category; they are diplomats and they care for everyone else before caring for themselves. Think about your own style and how it affects your ability to understand who you are and how you function. This will be critical as you evaluate your own reinvention process.

*"Passion is universal humanity. Without it religion, history, romance and art would be useless."*

*—Honoré de Balzac*

# HOW DO I KNOW WHEN ENOUGH IS ENOUGH?

Take a moment to reflect on your career. If you were to lose your job today, how would that affect you? If you needed a professional recommendation, who would you contact to provide it? How would that recommendation look and feel? Do others think of you as a resource, as a go-to person? You may love your work, but dislike those with whom you work. Work satisfaction studies reveal that job frustration is the number-one problem that people express. We have all experienced the typical bad day at the office, so when is enough just that—enough? I recommend listening to your body; it is a great indicator. If your job makes you ill, it might be time to look elsewhere.

Can you fix what is not working about your job? Can you change units, or move your desk to another location? Sometimes, even changing the position of your desk helps. Is there opportunity for professional growth and can you learn from this position and use that knowledge to advance your career?

What kind of work and work setting excite you? What would give you great joy in the workplace? Do you prefer to work alone, or as a part of a team? What steps have you taken thus far to change your situation, and what is your timeline for change? Put yourself in a position in which resignation is a good choice rather than a desperate one.

*"Be thankful for what you have; you'll end up having more. If you concentrate on what you don't have, you will never, ever have enough."*

*—Oprah Winfrey*

Why are you here today? Why are you reading this book? Are you over the hill like Charles Schultz, picking up speed, growing wiser or growing more careful like Hemingway? Have you been in your present position for a year, 2 years, or more? Are you in a dead-end position that seems to lack a future? Do you hate your boss, or are you the boss?

Is it time for you to reinvent yourself? I have done it several times. Growing up with parents who told me to learn to type because I would never amount to anything, I was challenged at an early age to be the best of the best. As the middle of five kids, I did not have the "middle child syndrome," but I did have the "caught in the middle syndrome," and, it was not fun! So, I started at an early age to identify ways in which I could better myself, learn and do more, achieve great heights, and then start all over again.

I entered nursing school because I liked people, got a scholarship from the Philadelphia public schools, and had a safe place to live. I loved patient care. I often thought that there were patients who could not possibly recover without my presence on each and every shift. I worked harder and smarter than many of my classmates, and I was a good student, albeit an impatient one. I was always in anticipation of the next step, the next part of the obstacle course, the next challenge.

As I think back, I realize that part of my wish to reinvent myself stemmed from a lack of self-esteem and an awareness that others were brighter and kinder than I was, and that they came from what seemed to be (at least on the outside) loving families. So, part of reinventing myself involved giving myself a new look, a new role, and a new career. I had an opportunity to shine beyond my wildest dreams, and I worked hard at it.

People reinvent themselves for different reasons. For some, it's the sudden realization that they're not happy or fulfilled. This is what's commonly called a midlife crisis. The reinventors, on the other hand, prefer the term "finding themselves," particularly when they're not in the mood to admit that they're flat-out bored and need a change. Some of you may have kids who are still finding themselves, or you may be that person yourself.

# Reinventing Yourself

"The fundamental quest at midlife is to figure out who we are and who we want to be as we get ready to embark on the second half of life," writes Goldstein (2011). Goldstein is right. Identity is a major concern for midlifers and for good reason.

Midlifers need permission to reinvent themselves. New times require new identities, and sometimes the old ones we thought were just fine were not really that good in the first place! As a child, did you please your parents, cover for their transgressions? As an adult, do you cover for your spouse when he wants to stay home, cover for your kids when they do not complete assignments? Do you need to be needed? Do you take the time to please yourself?

Are you a controller—do you have to be in command at home and at work? Are you a hands-on guy with a rigid agenda? When do we get to see the real you? Do you dream of greener pastures? Is there an "Acre of Diamonds" (Nightingale, 2002) out there just waiting for you? When you walk through your own scruffy yard, you see all of its imperfections up close—the brown spots, the holes, the weeds—but when you look at your neighbor's pasture, it appears to be as seamlessly and magnificently green as the best golf course on a dewy morning. When you assess your contribution to mankind, the job that you hold, the career that you have chosen, you realize that you are either sitting on a gold mine, or you need to locate one. Your true worth is great, but it remains unrealized until you find the courage to dig beneath the hard surface of your identity: the identity of supervisor, VP, director.

# THE IDENTITY CRISIS

In American society young professionals are taught to define themselves by what they do: "I teach at Kellogg." "I am a trader." "I am a Chicago lawyer." "I program computers." "I work for IBM." "I'm a senior vice president." As we grow older, work identity can become shallow or cease to exist completely. We hit a plateau and a once-exciting job starts to seem bland. Sometimes we get demoted or even laid off. It is a frightening thing to be unemployed when your identity is your job. "Who am I if I'm not a geologist for Exxon?" "What am I if not a senior vice president for Abbott Laboratories?"

The term "young professionals" includes working women, some of whom may be moms. Perhaps they aren't sure who they are when children move away. The empty-nest syndrome sets in. Women sometimes take time away from the workplace to raise a family, and reentry to the workforce (not unlike a spacecraft reentering the Earth's atmosphere) is intimidating at best. Plus, a society that focused on outward appearance has nothing to offer the aging female psyche. Barbara Fried sums up the anguish of many midlife women: "Everything that makes life worth living for me is either turning gray, drying up, or leaving home." Is that you?

# AN EXCITING ADVENTURE

Forging a new identity offers great promise. "A single fixed identity is a liability today," writes *New Passages* (1995, p. 71) author Gail Sheehy. "It only makes people more vulnerable to sudden changes in economic or personal conditions." So Sheehy advocates multiple identities for midlifers—identities that will not only explain what we do but who we are.

Many years ago, as inexperienced and fickle teenagers, most of us constructed our adult identities. We've lived with them now for between 10 and 30 years (or more), and we've done surprisingly well. Now it's time to reevaluate them in light of our changing world and time-acquired wisdom. It's time to reinvent a new us that will take us through our second adulthood. So who are you? Who do you want to be when you grow up (a question that my kids often ask of me)? This time, you get to decide.

Consider the following as you reinvent yourself:

1. **Keep your options open.** Don't turn down opportunities just because they are outside of the parameters of what you have thought to be your job title or place in life. The real opportunity might be behind a previously closed door. (Visit wiifYOU.com.)

2. **Cross-pollinate.** Take your knowledge, skills, and abilities from one field to another. Step outside your comfort zone. Look for ideas to bring into your field from others. Plant your ideas within entirely new fields, new pastures.

3. **Follow your heart's desire and your dream.** Your heart is a wise barometer of what you need to be doing with your life. Think from the heart as well as the mind when you evaluate opportunities.

4. **Live a little.** If you went to graduate school right out of university without taking time to experience life, do it now. Experience often prods us to do something beyond our wildest imaginations. The more experiences you accumulate, the more you get a view of what works for you and what doesn't.

5. **Visualize.** Paint a picture in your mind's eye of what you want in your life. I often print out the words, attach a photo, and hang it on my bulletin board. It is what I see in the morning when I enter my office, and what I see later in the day. It is a constant reminder of what I expect to achieve and what I believe is within my reach. Take every chance to experience this inner image with all of your five senses.

6. **Be curious.** Keep your eyes and ears open and your antenna up for new people and new ideas to enter your life. You have heard that it is not what you know, but who you know that counts. This has never been truer than in the field of reinvention.

7. **Network like crazy.** Make it a point to meet new people as often as you can. New people in your life will enrich you and lead you to new opportunities. Don't make networking experiences about you; listen actively to what others say in the networking community. Be a giver because givers gain.

8. **Within nursing, there is a theory known as novice to expert.** The theory evolved as the result of work by Dr. Patricia Benner (2013). She proposed that one could gain knowledge and skills ("knowing how") without ever learning the theory ("knowing that"). New nurses must begin as novices. They must learn skill sets that were not taught in school; for example, they must learn to communicate with patients, families, and other healthcare providers, and they must grow in expertise and experience. Although I have remained in the healthcare field, moving from intervention to prevention, I know that there is no limit to one's growth potential within a vastly changing industry. Be a student of continuous learning. Seek new ways to stretch yourself. Find new challenges to master. Attend classes and workshops.

9. **Embrace new ideas and technology.** They will prepare you for opportunity, growth, and the future.

As you consider these principles, consider trying the following things:

- Find a new pursuit that allows you to approach it as a beginner.
- Think that there are no bad jobs. It is the way in which we go about our work that makes it good or bad.
- Put your imagination to work on the many ways and means of improving what you are now doing. Our dynamic and growing economy needs and rewards the uncommon person who prepares for a place in its growth.
- Think about how you would reinvent yourself.

Think about traditional and alternative work/life patterns that you have experienced, or of which you are aware. In a traditional work setting, you have a job and a boss. Compare that traditional with alternative styles; think about what works for you. There may be positives and negatives in each column, but choose those that would bring joy and balance to your own life.

| Trading time for money, a.k.a. the traditional work/life pattern | Time and money freedom, a.k.a. the alternative work/life pattern |
|---|---|
| 1. Work for someone else and live for the weekends and holidays | 1. Work for yourself and set your own priorities on time and money |
| 2. Lack control of your own future | 2. Focus on personal and professional growth and enjoy new experiences |
| 3. Work to realize someone else's dream, rather than your own | 3. Remain happy and productive, with the knowledge that your Plan B will continue to provide for you |
| 4. Retire, perhaps on a pension if funds are still available, and worry about whether or not your funds will carry you through the rest of your life | 4. Eat well, keep physically fit, and enjoy being with others |
| 5. Experience declining emotional/physical/spiritual health and ask yourself, "Why?" | 5. Live a long and happy life, working the hours that you choose to work, enjoying new things and new people |

Think of the mouse in *Who Moved My Cheese* (1998), the adult parable made famous by Spencer Johnson. At some point in your life, you have to make a decision. You have to change. Change is a constant and an essential catalyst for reinventing ourselves, our lives, and our work. Change usually takes courage and tenacity, especially when there is no guarantee of success. Change is a process of reinvention. Chandler (2005) states that it is easy to get stuck in a humdrum life and fantasize about what could have been. You don't have to wait for middle age or be in the midst of a crisis to reinvent yourself. In fact, it's a lot more fun when you're neither. Keep in mind that if your reinvention doesn't work out, you can always reinvent yourself again.

# What Resources Are Available to You?

We live in the information age, and the opportunities are limitless. Career counseling, college resource centers, and other resources make the search and the process easier. What is more difficult to handle is the fact that there are thousands of applicants for even the most mundane positions. Consider career coaching with a certified professional.

# Professional Coaching

Professional coaching empowers you to be your best, feel your best, and do your best in your business and personal life and in your career search. By starting with your life's purpose and identifying what is important in your life, your goals are set, and you can begin the implementation process. Coaching works because you have an objective partner in the process; your coach helps you to reach the competitive edge that sets you apart from others and establishes you in your field. Your coach enhances your ability to solve your own problems with practical strategies that are action oriented, an accountability system that keeps you motivated, a fresh perspective to challenge your limiting beliefs, and support when you need it most. From platform skills to improved performance, a coach may lead the way.

# What Is It Like to Start Over?

Many people may feel that they are too old, or lack the education, money, or time to do what they really want to do. But that is not true. What *is* true is what, in your mind's eye, you see as possible. Look at where you are now and move toward that which you want to become. AARP offers wonderful resources for those third agers considering a career change or looking for a new job (http://www.aarp.org/money/work).

# Live an Intentional Life

As you continue to find balance, remember that whatever opportunities appear in your life, you are equipped to handle them and handle them well. Full participation on an emotional, physical, spiritual, and intellectual level enhances your life and that of those around you. Keep an open mind; be open to other areas of life to which you may not have been exposed. Create a calendar of places to go and people to see. This might include something you have been longing to do, or something that you perhaps thought about but never dared to do.

I often think of my nursing school roommate. A diploma graduate, she went on to obtain a bachelor's degree from the University of Pennsylvania and became a master's-prepared neonatal nurse specialist. Years later, as she traveled with her physician husband to new assignments, she lost her passion for nursing, but not for people. She opened an antique shop in a small town and has enjoyed tremendous success. Now, in her next reinvention, she is a deaconess of the church.

*"Each decision we make, each action we take, is born out of an intention."*

—Sharon Salzberg

Sometimes our identities get lost or buried over the years, and we realize we have not done the things that we always dreamed of doing, such as traveling, starting our own wellness business, or building a community around a tea café. It is important to visualize those things by writing them down and revisiting the thoughts that you left behind. You may ask yourself, "Is it possible to resurrect my current position and inject life into it?"

## ARE THERE GREENER PASTURES?

Are there greener pastures (and I do not mean farming)? Does the grass always look greener on the other side of the fence? In the classic *Lead the Field* (2002), Earl Nightingale addresses the subject of greener pastures. Sometimes the greener pasture is the one in which you currently sit; it may be in your own backyard.

## SHARE THE PASSION

Regardless of your particular career choice or situation, it is hard to maintain a level of passion about your life when those around you don't feel the same, particularly in the workplace. There are always other people who have been in dead-end jobs themselves, maybe for many years. Or, some of your colleagues may dislike what they do; don't have a defined purpose for being; feel inadequate, underpaid, unloved, unappreciated, and myriad other feelings that you can probably understand yourself. Don't let those around you drag you down, particularly when you've worked hard to balance or rebalance your life. Don't stoop to their level of unhappiness! Don't feel less passionate about what you are doing because others do not value it! Do see the opportunity to rise to the occasion and lead by example. Rather than try to explain to others how you are feeling and what you are doing, show them with your actions. When you are joyous and productive in your daily life others will observe that and be curious.

*"There is nothing like returning to a place that remains unchanged to find the ways in which you yourself have altered."*

*–Nelson Mandela*

I still recall a class reunion where I was the only one present without a walker, cane, or wheelchair. I knew the ages of my classmates. We had, after all, started our education together at ages 17 or 18. My colleagues asked me what I had been doing that allowed me to be in so much better physical shape than they were. They assumed that it was some sort of miracle drug that had given me a new lease on life. Frankly, I did not need a new lease because the old one had not yet run out. My good health was my passion! And, my passion related to my newfound interest in health and wellness, as opposed to disease and sickness. I'll admit that part of this interest came with being a new grandparent and my desire to sit on the floor and play…and be able to get up again. I demonstrated, through my actions, a passion for wellness and overall well-being.

I remember when one of my colleagues asked if I had my knees replaced yet. I replied that the originals were still working, and I did not plan to replace them simply because I had reached a certain age.

# Finding and Sharing Your Bliss

Invite others to share in what you do in your life that is making such a difference. By including other people in your activities they are more likely to be open to the changes you are experiencing in your life. People around you will respond to your efforts in showing them what you are learning and discovering.

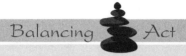

## FIND AND SHARE YOUR BLISS

- Set aside time for yourself every day. This can be a quiet time that you schedule into your day, every day. Use this time to think, write, read, meditate or do anything else that will further your passions. Those around you will adjust quickly to this time and will not interrupt you. It is your time to be, and to appreciate, you.

- Focus on what you love, eliminating as much as possible that does not feed your joy or energy.

- Go with your feelings and emotions and do what feels good! So many of us have allowed others to tell us what we should do, think, and feel for so long that it might take some time for you to find your bliss. Stick with it, and the world will be at your command.

# WHEN OPPORTUNITY KNOCKS, ANSWER

We are in a never-ending state of change. We are constantly growing and evolving, and it is impossible to remain the same person you are today even if you wanted to. Think about your own career and the number of times that you have reinvented yourself.

*"Not knowing when the dawn will come, I open every door."*

*—Emily Dickinson*

When you started your career, chances are that you did not immediately envision yourself as the chief operating officer. Chances are that you thought of yourself as a staff worker, clinician, or perhaps as a future educator helping to mold the minds and spirits of the next generation. Your aspirations related to the next step or two in front of you. At some point in your career, though, you chose a specialty and developed your skills to a level of being the best that you could be in your field—an expert. You may have become involved in leadership initiatives within your organization, maybe even became part of an elite team working on Magnet initiatives, shared governance models, or internal councils. Perhaps you joined a professional group and assumed a leadership role within that organization. If a local chapter was within your field of vision, you may have started it. If a national position was within your field of vision, perhaps you took the steps necessary and paid your dues along the way to make that a reality.

*"Change is the constant, the signal for rebirth, the egg of the phoenix."*

—Christina Baldwin

Don't' be afraid to challenge yourself. You never know where a new experience may take you. For example, I was working in an emergency department in a community hospital before I began my infusion specialty practice. A patient arrived in acute distress and needed an intravenous infusion. I had never performed that procedure. I wasn't even trained in it. The emergency department physician challenged me to start the infusion, and after consulting the procedure manual and the product label, I started the infusion successfully. It was at that moment that I decided to become the best that I could be, and to learn all that I could about the practice of infusion nursing. From that moment of inspiration, I became a local and national leader, national president, director of the certification board, and author of the textbook that I initially read back in 1975. I reinvented myself as an infusion specialist, and I continue to evolve in my career today with a focus on medical safety and fatigue.

# WHAT ARE THE OPPORTUNITIES

From a small business to a franchise, from a network marketing career to a project development consulting practice, opportunities abound.

By knowing yourself, by assessing your skill sets, by understanding the thought process, you can distinguish what is needed to succeed.

# How Will I Know?

This question applies to all aspects of our lives. How will you know when you have met the right "one"? How will you know if the offer is a good one? How will you know if it is time to move on, and if the fit at the new job is right? If you lack passion and are miserable each morning, it is time to go. If you are stressed, feel ill, and dislike your coworkers, it is time to go. If the corporate culture is not a good match and you lack work/life balance, it is time to go. If you have no "voice" and you lack meaningful recognition, it is time to go. The important thing is that you have evaluated your options, considered your reinvention, and are not making an emotional decision.

# Entrepreneurship

Entrepreneurs have a term for outsized problems they want to tackle or bigger-than-life bets they want to make: *moon shots*. Examples include Google's driverless cars and Amazon's delivery-by-drone. Entrepreneurship is now taught at major universities across the nation and around the world. The concept has moved beyond the business school to the high-school classroom.

There is something to be said for building your own dream rather than someone else's dream. Is the best entrepreneur one who is a persistent visionary or a highly reactive opportunist? There is more than one right answer, and there are many paths to becoming an entrepreneur. A consulting practice that started as Plan B may become so busy that it becomes Plan A. A part-time position in direct sales or network marketing may become so successful that you realize that you must leave your day job in order to maintain work/life balance. The qualities that make a good entrepreneur include resilience, the ability to take feedback, having the courage of your convictions, an innate belief in your product/service/ability, hard work, and focus. Entrepreneurs are those who grow great ideas. If this describes you, get out there and start growing!

# NETWORKING

You have certainly heard that it is not what you know, but who you know that counts. Use this opportunity to build your LinkedIn profile and to make it shine. Ask for recommendations from those with whom you have worked and have those recommendations posted on your behalf. Ask for connections to others who are not in your network but who work for companies in which you have an interest.

Many chambers of commerce and professional groups have special meetings for those who are in transition or between success stories. Take advantage of those opportunities to connect with others.

# AGE IS NO OBSTACLE

Age is just a number. It is time to think of yourself as a seasoned professional! There is never a bad time to reinvent your life, no matter how early or late it is in your career. You can do anything you want to do at any time. Did you know that there's a movement for established career types called the "*third age*"? The third age is a life stage created by life expectancies that reach into the 80s and beyond—a time that represents new possibilities for living in fulfillment and purpose. Third agers are typically anywhere between 45 and 65, have raised their children, and face many healthy, productive years left in their lives. These are people who may need to move out of a physically demanding job—such as bedside nurses or product line workers—but plan to work for a number of years before retiring, or they may be retirees who need to—or choose to—return to work for income, personal enrichment, or social reasons.

"Human beings have an inalienable right to invent themselves."

—Germaine Greer

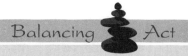

## DOWN MEMORY LANE

You have the power to reinvent yourself at any point in your life. Age, position, job, circumstances: None of these should stand in your way. Think about how quickly Thanksgiving dinner turns into conversations that begin, "Hey, remember when we...." Those stories are often about things that we recall imperfectly, that may or may not have happened, or that others remember differently, but, it remains great fun to share the stories as well as the memories. It is like a walk down memory lane. In a personal development program, I participated in a game called "Down Memory Lane." The concept was to remember yourself as a small child and to think about what brought you satisfaction in life, what may have frightened you, and your responses.

Take time to walk down memory lane. Write down what brought you great satisfaction—that is what you want to focus on as you move forward in life. Write down what brought you the least satisfaction and avoid those situations as much as possible!

*"We cannot change what we are not aware of, and once we are aware, we cannot help but change."*

*–Sheryl Sandberg*

# AFFIRMATIONS

You have a full caseload, a full workweek, family responsibilities, and more obligations! You have the power within to change lives each and every day of your career. We all need interaction and affirmation in our lives. I have made a daily habit of stating and repeating affirmations aloud that support my passion for being. For example, I might say, "Today someone somewhere will benefit from my act of kindness."

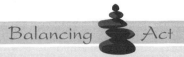

Balancing Act

## PRACTICE A DAILY PLAN FOR REINVENTION

Every day is a new beginning and an opportunity to reinvent oneself. Begin with 10 to 20 minutes of meditation or quiet time. Picture yourself living the life of your dreams. This can be difficult sometimes because we are so caught up with the reality of our daily lives. But don't let reality get in the way of your dreams. Whatever you think about and picture in your mind's eye you are capable of manifesting into your life.

We are indeed spiritual beings living a physical experience, not the other way around. Expect miracles from your life every day. Remember that everything in our material world was once someone's abstract dream. If we did not dream for the future we would not have the things that we give so much value to today.

What about you? As a professional, your own priorities are usually not about you. When do you have time to debrief? When do you take the time to encourage others to pursue a life's dream? Think about and identify your core values, prioritize your needs, and then dream the big dream. Is this the right time to reinvent yourself and your career? Think of those who have done it successfully and be willing to know the real you! You can do it as no one else can.

So step back, look at the big picture, and use your perspective to help people feel good about themselves; that is the critical skill that's allowed me to touch the lives of others on a global scale! I can combine my background in western medicine with integrative and functional medicine to help people feel better and live longer naturally. From personal experience, I know that sometimes the quality of our well-being comes down to the environment in which we live and work. That environment can hinder our ability to be well and can create stress-induced illness. This can take a huge toll on energy levels and the feeling of well-being we all rely on to have optimal vitality and wellness.

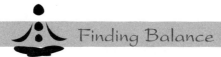

## Finding Balance

## REFLECTIONS

- Things change, including us.
- We are constantly in process.
- Reflect on yourself and your achievements.
- Treat yourself with kindness.

# REFERENCES

Benner, P. (2013). Nursing theories: From novice to expert. Retrieved from http://currentnursing.com/nursing_theory/Patricia_Benner_From_Novice_to_Expert.html

Chandler, S. (2005). *Reinventing yourself: How to become the person you've always wanted to be* (revised edition). New Jersey: The Career Press.

Chen, H. (2011). *The 5 elements of success.* Richmond, BC: Alphay. Retrieved from http://www.alphayglobal.com/portals/0/pdf/five_elements_of_success.pdf

Cunningham, L. (2012, December 14). Does it pay to know your type? The Myers-Briggs Type Indicator. *The Washington Post.* Retrieved from http://www.washingtonpost.com/business/on-leadership/myers-briggs-does-it-pay-to-know-your-type/2012/12/14/eaed51ae-3fcc-11e2-bca3-aadc9b7e29c5_story.html

Goldstein, R. E. (2011). *Chain reaction.* CreateSpace Independent Publishing Platform.

Johnson, S. (1998). *Who moved my cheese?* New York: Penguin Group.

Nightingale, E. (2002, first published in 1986). *Lead the field.* New York: Simon and Schuster.

Sheehy, G. (1995). *New passages: Mapping your life across time.* New York: Random House.

"I seldom end up where I wanted to go, but almost always end up where I need to be."

–Douglas Adams

# 12

# DESTINY IN THE BALANCE

*–Sharon M. Weinstein, MS, RN, CRNI, FACW, FAAN*

In the end, the key word is balance. You need to find the right balance that works for you. Celebrate your successes and don't dwell on your failures. Life is a process, and so is striving for balance in your life. A universal law that is the basis of all economic and personal well-being describes how to put the law to work for you, increase your effectiveness, and experience a more abundant life.

We all assume many roles in life—roles in the family, in the workplace, in the physical community, and in the professional community. Each role enables us to express a different dimension of our being. It is these separate roles that need to be balanced in our lives. For example, your life needs balancing if you are professionally successful but your family complains that you do not spend enough time with them. Your lifestyle needs balancing if, again, your career is soaring but your health is challenged. Finally, if you are addicted to a favorite TV show but have no time to clean your closets or the garage, then your life needs balancing.

"Gather only what you need; travel lightly, and keep moving forward. The journey will be more joyful with less baggage."

—Deborah Haggerty

# ATTITUDE

Your destiny lies in achieving balance, and there are two major ways in which to balance your life. Because life coexists with time, the first way to balance life is to balance time. Many outstanding publications address time management, some of which are specific to nursing professionals. Find the ones that suit your style and needs, and use them! The second way to balance life is by balancing your attitude. An attitude of gratitude is critical to success in life. Some call it a winning or a positive attitude. Everything flows from it. Basically, things work best for those who make the best of the way things work out.

"At times our own light goes out and is rekindled by a spark from another person. Each of us has cause to think with deep gratitude of those who have lighted the flame within us."

—Albert Schweitzer

Many years ago, a large American shoe manufacturer sent two sales representatives to different parts of the Australian outback to see if they could generate business among the aboriginal people. Some time later, the company received messages from both agents. The first one said, "No business here; natives don't wear shoes." The second one said, "Great opportunity here; natives don't wear shoes." If you can't change your fate—if you can't see a market for shoes among people who don't wear them—change your attitude.

"A positive attitude turns 'I can't & I won't,' into 'I have and I will.'"

—Mandy Hale

Although we all would like to be successful, many people have reasons upon reasons why they cannot succeed. In truth, all we need to succeed is one reason why we *can*. That reason is attitude. Nothing is more important—not education, aptitude, health, wealth, or opportunity.

What is *attitude*? Attitude is our disposition, perspective, viewpoint, or outlook. It is how we view the world. If we perceive the glass as half full, it is; if we perceive it as half empty, it is. That is, we don't see things as they are; we see things as we are—we interpret our experiences, labeling them as good or bad. However, our interpretations do not affect reality; they just affect us.

## Balancing Act

### SMILE THERAPY

It may seem or feel silly at first, but challenge yourself to smile at everyone you meet for one full day. Don't worry if they don't smile back. Just keep smiling. By the end of the day, you'll be happier as smiling creates energy whereas frowning takes energy.

Some people, for instance, love cold weather; others hate it. Obviously, our feelings have no influence on the temperature, as no matter how angry or grumpy we get about the cold temperature, it won't get warmer. I, for one, would love to live in an area in which the temperature range was 50 to 75 degrees Fahrenheit. However, that would impact my balance, because I would be too far from those near and dear to me.

Our emotions have great effect on our lives, bringing us happiness or unhappiness. Some of us can discover opportunity in every difficulty; others find nothing but difficulty in every opportunity—same circumstances, but different perspective, thus different attitudes.

"We shall never know all the good that a simple smile can do."

—Mother Teresa

One way to change your life is to change your attitude. You might be asking, "How do I change my attitude?" It's simple, really; just behave the way you want to become. Are you a pessimist who wishes to become an optimist? If so, pretend to be optimistic. When you change your behavior, you change everything within your worldview. At first, it might feel forced, but the longer you do it, the more it becomes a habit—a positive habit—that will be just as easy to live in as your old pessimistic patterns. The world is a mirror, so behave as if you are happy. When you do that, the world will reflect back happiness. Be downcast, and the world responds similarly. It is not the position, but the *disposition* that makes this possible. Learn to be grateful for what you already have; think of the life that you have and how blessed you already are—then value it! Also be thankful for what you have while you pursue all that you want in life.

"We who lived in concentration camps can remember the men who walked through the huts comforting others, giving away their last piece of bread. They may have been few in number, but they offer sufficient proof that everything can be taken from a man but one thing: the last of the human freedoms—to choose one's attitude in any given set of circumstances, to choose one's own way."

—Victor Frankl

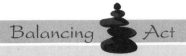

### THE POWER OF POSITIVE THINKING

- Use positive action words when talking and thinking. Words like "I can" and "I will" are powerful and help support attitude change. Carry this through into all your conversations.

- Push out all feelings that aren't positive. Don't let negative thoughts and feelings overwhelm you when you're feeling down. Even if it's only for a few hours a day, push your negativity aside and focus only on the good things in your life.

- Surround yourself with positive people.

- Before starting with any plan or action, visualize clearly in your mind its successful outcome. If you visualize with concentration and faith, you will be amazed at the results.

- Always sit and walk with your back straight. This will strengthen your confidence and inner strength.

# MIND-SET

Your mind-set is everything; it will make or break you. Mind-set is a set of assumptions, methods, or notations held by one or more people that drive behavior, choices, and outcomes. Strive to balance and integrate the physical, emotional, mental, and spiritual aspects of your life. Establish respectful, cooperative relationships with your family, friends, community, and the environment. Gather information and make informed, wellness-oriented choices. Actively participate in your own health decisions and healing process. Crum and Langer (2007) studied whether the relationship between exercise and health is moderated by one's mind-set. They were able to demonstrate that exercise affects health in part or in whole.

Think about it—you are your own team! The *physical* you requires good nutrition, healthy weight, beneficial exercise, and adequate rest. The *emotional* you needs to give and receive forgiveness, love, and compassion; it needs to laugh and experience happiness; and it needs joyful relationships between yourself and others. The *mental* you needs self-supportive attitudes, positive thoughts and viewpoints, and a positive self-image. The *spiritual* you requires inner calmness, openness to your creativity, and trust in your inner knowing. A comfortable, healthy balance between your physical, mental, emotional, and spiritual aspects doesn't happen accidentally. It is purposeful; someone has to be in charge, and that someone is always you. Have a growth mind-set—one in which you are consistently open to new ideas, to continuous learning, and to self-improvement. Make the internal dialogue with yourself a positive one as you pursue your goals.

*"We like to think of our champions and idols as superheroes who were born different from us. We don't like to think of them as relatively ordinary people who made themselves extraordinary."*

—Carol S. Dweck

# CHANGE YOUR MIND AND CHANGE YOUR LIFE

As founder of the International Nursing Leadership Institute hosted by the American International Health Alliance (AIHA), I had the opportunity to collaborate with many nurse leaders as we shared knowledge and expertise with our peers from the new independent States of the former Soviet Union and Central and Eastern European nations. We made the learning process fun through role play, modeling the behaviors of the characters and enjoying the learning process. Our goal was to create a cadre of nurse leaders/educators. Faculty used a series of leading management books to generate the curriculum. Language barriers were a challenge, so students and faculty, in full costume, acted out the stories. For example, the parable *Who Moved My Cheese?* (Johnson, 1998) encouraged students to have contingency plans and to expect change.

*Who Moved My Cheese?* captures that moment we may have experienced at some point in our own lives, perhaps after we have lost a job or a relationship and we believe it is the end of the world. Fear overwhelms us as we ponder the future. Everything we had was great (even if we did not enjoy the job). Yet the author encourages us to see change as a beginning, rather than an end. Does that sound familiar? I'll bet it does. We realize that change happens, and we need to be prepared to evaluate, value, and implement the change. Change is inevitable. Focus on changing your mind and changing your life. First you must understand change in order to be open to the process and realize the effects.

# THE FIVE ELEMENTS: FINDING THE FIVE ELEMENTS WITHIN YOU

Chapter 2 discusses *5 Elements of Success* (Chen, 2011), Hui Chen's ebook about what is important in life and how that may be used to build a balanced existence. The philosophy of Five Elements extends beyond that vision to include nature. In ancient Chinese medicine, also known as Traditional Chinese Medicine (TCM), we are exposed to the belief that there is a balance in the universe that forms all physical, elemental and dimensional relationships. The harmony that balance creates is something that is constantly sought in all matters of life. And after it is achieved, all health, personal purpose, and spiritual evolution will fall into place.

The Chinese believe there are five seasons: Fall, Winter, Spring, Summer (the four we commonly discuss), and Late Summer, which I affectionately refer to as "Cold and Flu Season." Behind each of the seasons there is an elemental energy created by Wood, Fire, Earth, Water, or Metal. By being aware of nature we can see these five energies in the world around us and also see how these same energies are reflected within our own bodies and personalities. The Elements represent the transformation that occurs in the world around us; they are metaphors for describing how things interact and relate with each other. When they are balanced, we, too, are balanced. Think about your own personality style and relate it to mind, body, family, society, and finances.

Know that many caregivers, health professionals, and woman are Earth personalities. They take care of others before caring for themselves. Does that sound familiar, and could your style be a cause of imbalance in your own life? The following examines the relationship between key facets of life important to us all, the 5 Elements, and the personality style they represent.

- **Mind:** Wood (organized, mindful, innovative)
- **Body:** Fire (energetic, expressive)
- **Family:** Earth (trustful, loyal, responsible)
- **Society:** Water (resourceful, smart)
- **Finances:** Metal (determined, disciplined)

## THE VISION BOARD

What is a vision board, why should you have one, and how is it used? A vision board is a visual display of what you value in life. Your vision (yes, even in the form of a board or diagram) is the blueprint for your success. Why is it critical to have a plan at the start of a new year? How many times have you made a resolution that was broken by January 15th? When you surround yourself with images of who you want to become, what you want to have, where you want to live or vacation, your life changes to match those images and those desires. How do you begin? Gather your materials, identify your *why*, know your purpose, and then create your vision.

*"Gratitude makes sense of our past, brings peace for today, and creates a vision for tomorrow."*

*—Melody Beattie*

## CREATING A VISION BOARD

1. Gather magazines and download photos or clippings from the Internet that inspire you.

2. Collect favorite family photos, especially those in which you are included.

3. Select a background paper or board. I suggest an 8½" x 20" piece that you can fold and carry with you everywhere. Mine is in a plastic sheet protector, but it is always with me.

4. Assemble a glue stick, scissors, and your imagination.

5. Arrange the photos and inspirational quotes according to your interests. Mine are Personal and Professional Growth (Mind), Family, Society, Health, and Finances.

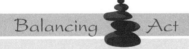

Balancing Act

## FINDING YOUR ELEMENTS BY FINDING JOY IN YOUR LIFE

With the Five Elements of Life in mind, ask yourself these questions:

- What are the three things in life that bring me the greatest joy?

- What am I willing to give up so that I can experience that joy on a continuous basis?

*"Without joy in your life, you are powerless."*

*—Joyce Meyers*

Remember, everyone is unique. It is unreasonable to expect to perfectly balance each role in life. Further, there will be times where you focus more on one aspect of life than another. The important lesson is not about balancing your life perfectly, but about balancing it in a manner that best expresses your potential and that gives you the most health and joy. You do this by adhering to the rule of *BE…DO…HAVE*.

You have to *BE* self-disciplined to *DO* what is needed to balance your life; when you do so, you will *HAVE* balance in the five facts of life known as mind, body, family, society, and finances.

# CHANGE BEGINS WITH CHOICE

All people have and make choices; these choices affect our lives in many ways. Being aware of the change process and how you adapt to change facilitates a life in balance.

## CHANGE HAPPENS

Everything in life is a choice. You have chosen the life you are living right now. You move toward your life's purpose, following your dreams, and are forced to make choices along the way. This is life's greatest truth and most difficult lesson. It is what gives you the power to be yourself and to live the life you imagined. Don't allow self-doubt to interfere with your success. Had I done that as a young girl, I would not be where I am now. There is no such thing as an impossible dream; there are only dreams without action steps to make it a reality. Go ahead and dream those lofty dreams—you shall become them!

*"Sometimes the dreams that come true are the dreams you never even knew you had."*

—Alice Sebold

## Shifting Paradigms

Any day you want, you can discipline yourself to change it all. Any day you want, you can read the book that will open your mind to new knowledge. Any day you want, you can start a new activity. Any day you want, you can start the process of life change. You can do it immediately, next week, next month, or next year. You can also do nothing, but you wouldn't be reading this book if you were looking for that choice.

Consider the following options (which we mentioned earlier in the book) as you seek destiny in the balance:

1. **Keep your options open.** Don't turn down opportunities just because they are outside the parameters of what you have thought to be your job title or place in life. The real opportunity might be behind a previously closed door.

2. **Cross-pollinate.** Take your knowledge, skills, and abilities from one field to another. Step outside your comfort zone. Look for ideas to bring into your field from others. Plant your ideas within entirely new fields, new pastures.

3. **Follow your heart's desire and live your passion.** Your heart is a wise barometer of what you need to be doing with your life. Think from the heart as well as the mind when you evaluate opportunities. Don't live by the dreams of others. Rather, live your own dreams.

4. **Live a little.** If you went to graduate school right out of university without taking time to experience life, do it now. Experience often prods us to do something beyond our wildest imaginations. The more experiences you accumulate, the more you get a view of what works for you and what doesn't. These experiences provide the basis for ongoing reinventions of self.

5. **Visualize.** Paint a picture in your mind's eye of what you want in your life. Don't underestimate the possibilities; think big and beautiful. I use this technique as a constant reminder of what I expect to achieve and what I believe is within my reach. Take every chance to experience this inner image with all of your five senses. (See the section about vision boards earlier in this chapter.)

6. **Be curious.** Keep your eyes and ears open and your antenna up for new people and new ideas to enter your life. You have heard that it is not what you know, but who you know that counts. This has never been truer than in the field of reinvention, and especially as we explore social media marketing and the use of technology.

7. **Network with like-minded people.** Make a point to meet new people as often as you can. New people in your life will enrich you and lead you to new opportunities. Don't make it about you; listen actively to what others say in the networking community. Be a giver because givers gain.

## CHANGING PRACTICE

Regardless of the type of work or industry, change happens. It may be clinical practice (think about how your own practice may have changed since your initial training); it may be technology, robotics, or something else. As the banking industry changed to automatic teller machines, we saw a significant decrease in the number of "live" tellers. There were fewer people working in banks, and there were fewer people going inside.

As the automotive and other industries became more automated, there has been less need for manual labor. As smart meters and other devices to measure utilization of power become more prominent, there will be fewer meter readers and more monitoring "in the cloud."

Are these sorts of changes in work process a good thing? Yes, they are, but it is how we perceive the changes, and how involved we become in adopting and implementing the changes that ensure success, acceptance, and growth.

## CREATING YOUR FUTURE

*"Bless not only the road but the bumps on the road.
They are all part of the higher journey."*

—Julia Cameron

We may have all grown up the same way, perhaps with the same advice from our parents. Get an education, get a job, and you will be rewarded for the rest of your life. You will be secure! We may have seen this model of success within our families with moms and dad who worked for the same company forever and then enjoyed a pension and retirement. They may have lived by the 40-40-40 rule: work 40 hours a week for 40 years and earn $40,000 annually! Times have changed, and so has the rule.

The 40-40-40 rule no longer works because the world is changing too quickly. Innovators are leading the change that we see in the world—innovators like the late, great Apple founder Steve Jobs. We have an opportunity to create our future, to transform our practice, to be the change we wish to see in the world. We can lead sustainability, environmental causes, and global action. The future holds economic disparities, aging populations, increasing global competition, and climate change. And yet, we can be prepared by being aware, becoming more educated, and by making choices in the face of fear.

# Keep Your Habits, but Change Your Choices

In my own practice, I coach others about the choices they make. Healthy living doesn't happen at the physician's or licensed independent practitioner's office. The road to better health is paved with the small decisions we make every day. It's about the choices we make when we buy groceries, drive our cars, and hang out with our kids. It's about our fast food stops, inhaling our food "on the run," and time constraints that prevent us from living a healthy lifestyle. When all of the systems within our complex bodies are in sync, we are balanced and charged. Think about the cell phone, PDA, or other assistive device that you use on a daily basis. When the charge is gone, what do you do? You simply plug it into an outlet or USB port and recharge the battery!

What about your most vulnerable human commodity: the body? What do you do when your cells are tired, toxic, thirsty, or just plain worn out?

First, you find the root cause, which might be lack of sleep, poor nutrition, dehydration, or burning the candle at both ends. That lifestyle may have worked well for you at age 20 or 30 (it did for me), but after a while, our bodies just do not respond well to abuse. So, what is a human body to do?

We have a choice in what we choose and in how we live. Yet we also have habits, many of which are unhealthy and have affected the overall health of our population. When we make decisions repeatedly, those decisions become our habits. (Read more about this in Chapter 2.) We no longer need to make a choice simply because we have habits—both good and bad. We may want to alter our habits, but we all know that life has a way of getting in the way. To form a new habit (a new choice) takes time, and time is the last thing that we have. What can we do? We can first be aware of our habits because we cannot change that of which we are unaware. Think about your own habits. Do you read books online or in hard copy? Do you sit in front of a computer screen all day? Do you consume lots of processed foods? After you've examined your choices then you can work on changing them. Yes, continue to drink coffee, but make it a healthier choice. Yes, continue to eat whole foods, but add consumables that are vegan, gluten-free, and organic. Eventually, good choices become good habits, and you are well on the way to a life in balance.

"No trumpets sound when the important decisions of our life are made. Destiny is made known silently."

—Agnes de Mille

At some point in your life, you have to make a decision. You have to change. Change is a constant, an essential catalyst for reinventing ourselves, our lives, and our work. Change usually takes courage and tenacity, especially when there is no guarantee of success. Change is a process of reinvention.

## OUT OF THE MOUTHS OF BABES

In his book, *Career Reexplosion: Reinvent Yourself in Thirty Days* (2000), Gary Joseph Grappo suggests that changing your career can change your life. To arrive at three new career directions to explore, he suggests this simple exercise:

- List at least 10 childhood experiences, situations, events, hobbies, interests, skills, education, and so on that you enjoyed and that made you happy.

- Repeat this list for activities that have made you happy throughout your adult years.

- Place these lists side by side and list your top ten dream careers that may be derived from the dreams, passions, and experiences you have accumulated from the two lists. Brainstorm with those you respect most, conduct an Internet search, and create the career of your vision and dreams without worrying about the education, money, or resources you'd need to achieve them.

- Narrow your wish list to the top three reinvention choices, keeping in mind they will be fluid and subject to change. Then, take action toward them and watch what happens. Reinvention is about a decision, a commitment, and action steps in support of that decision. Make the decision yours and yours alone.

# BALANCING WITH THE BEST OF THEM

The core of a balanced life is congruence with your values, dreams, and goals. How your life balances is up to you. You are the driver of your own bus! After you have determined where you are out of balance and how to rebalance, you will be primed to succeed like never before. Make a positive attitude an integral part of everything you do, and you will succeed faster than you ever imagined.

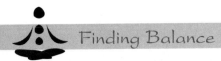
Finding Balance

## PRINCIPLES OF GOOD HEALTH

This final exercise helps you get ready to apply the principles you have learned in all aspects of your daily life.

Make three columns on a page; then write what you want to be, *do*, or *have* in each of the following categories:

HEALTHY BODY

HEALTHY MIND

HEALTHY FAMILY

HEALTHY SOCIETY

HEALTHY WORKPLACE

Now develop a plan to achieve your goals. Be sure to take small steps. For example, start with just one small goal in one area and let success build your confidence as you move from one area to the next.

## REFLECTIONS

- Living a balanced life is an ongoing and dynamic process.

- It requires change and change involves choice.

- Take control and take charge of your life now.

- Think about it; your new choices become your actions, actions become habits, and the new habits become your character.

- Yes, you can change your life and your destiny.

## REFERENCES

Chen, H. (2011). *The 5 elements of success.* Richmond, BC: Alphay. Retrieved from http://www.alphayglobal.com/portals/0/pdf/five_elements_of_success.pdf

Crum, A. J., & Langer, E. J. (2007). Mind-set matters: Exercise and the placebo effect. *Psychological Science, 18*(2), 165-171.

Grappo, G. (2000). *Career reexplosion: Reinvent yourself in 30 days.* New York: Putnam.

Johnson, S. (1998). *Who moved my cheese?* New York: Penguin Group.

# Appendix

# 26 Principles of Life

1. **All Are Related:** There is a Native American saying that translates roughly to "All are related." Everything in the universe is part of The Great Spirit, from a rock, to a plant, to a fish, to a human. The spirit flows between and within us all, and it is the building block of everything. Because we are all part of the same whole, we should treat the rest of the whole as if it is part of us—that is, with compassion and love. We are all part of the Great Spirit, just like all the different leaves on a tree are part of the tree.

2. **The Energy Flow:** The universe is composed of energy. This energy flows between everything and within us all. When we have internal blocks, the energy fails to flow correctly, causing illness, lethargy, and other symptoms. This energy can be directed consciously; we can see it and feel it. How we feel affects our energy levels. Negativity drains energy; positivity creates energy.

3. **We Are Beings of Both Spirit and Flesh:** We are spirits, but at the same time we are creatures of the flesh. We inhabit both worlds simultaneously, even though we are often unaware of it. We should not shun the flesh for spirit or vice versa. Both are equally important. We have to walk with one foot in each of these worlds and pay attention to both. Neglecting either world causes distress in the other.

4. **No One Entity Is Superior to Another:** No one being or creature is any better or greater than another. We are all the same. We are all on different paths and have different levels of understanding, but that does not make any one of us better than another. Humans are not masters of nature, animals, or plants. They are our companions and coinhabitants of this planet. We are not superior to them, nor do we own them. We should treat them all with respect.

5. **Belief Creates:** How we perceive the universe is shaped by our beliefs. If we believe we are in a hurry, then everyone else appears to be going slow. Through belief and positive thought, we can create virtually anything. We should believe in our abilities and ourselves, and we will succeed. We can combine the power of belief with visualization to bring anything into reality.

6. **Intuition:** Inside us, a voice speaks and guides us. It is our intuition. We can choose to ignore it or to listen to it. When we are in tune with our intuition and start to listen to it, we will be guided and will find that we can achieve more than we thought possible. We will begin to realize that the Great Spirit works through us—often in mysterious ways, but always to our benefit—in the long term.

7. **The Higher Purpose:** Everything that happens is for a reason and for the greater good. We have to learn to look at events in our lives from more than just the normal human perspective. We must see them from the perspective of the Great Spirit and to look at what good will come from these events. This is like the old maxim: "Is the glass half full or half empty?" We can look at events negatively (the half-empty perspective), and our reaction will be poor. However, when we look at events better (the half-full perspective) then we are more positive, which means our energy is higher, and our reaction will be better.

8. **There Are No Ordinary Moments:** The past only exists in our memory. The future only exists as our expectation. The only time that really exists is *now*. It is a precious moment, and we should treat every single moment as special and live it to the full. By being in the present, we have presence. To live in the now, your conscious mind should be quiet, and you must focus totally on what you are doing,

not what you are going to be doing next week, or what you are going to have for lunch.

9. **There Are No Limits:** The only limits we have are those we place upon ourselves or that others place upon us. To this end, we should avoid being put in a pigeonhole and labelled by others. If someone views a dog as being vicious then it is more likely to be vicious. We should hold no expectations of others, and let them be themselves, just as we should be ourselves.

10. **Action, Not Reaction:** We should be at a state where we do not react in a situation, but act. Reaction is unconscious, whereas action is conscious. We should not let past influences affect our actions. For example, if you were once bitten by a dog, when you next meet a dog, you should not let the past bite affect how you act toward dogs. There are times to act, as well as times to be still. By living in the present and having control of the conscious mind, we can better direct our action.

11. **Positivity Rules:** Negative thoughts attract negative events and drain our energy. Positive thoughts attract positive events and increase our energy. To this end, we should look at our thoughts and the events that happen to us in a positive light, realizing negative thoughts for what they are and releasing them.

12. **Posture, Pose, and Breathing:** Energy flows through the body as it flows through all things. If your posture and pose are bad, the energy cannot flow cleanly, which causes blockages that manifest as pain or illness. You breathe in energy from the world around you. Therefore, your breaths should be deep and full, coming from the bottom of the belly, not the chest. This enables you to maximize your energy. Deep breathing helps relax you. When you are stressed, angry, or afraid, your breathing changes to be shallower and faster. By consciously controlling your breathing and keeping it deep and even, you can release the stress, anger, or fear, enabling you to act consciously in the situation.

13. **Everything in Balance:** The universe exists in a state of balance, as should we. We can do anything we wish, but we should always do it to moderation, never to excess. When we do things to excess,

they can become addictive, which drains energy and may become negative. Being balanced allows us to act better in situations. If we straddle the fence, so to speak, we can jump off either way should we desire to.

14. **Intent Is Action:** You can intend to do anything, and your intent is important. However, unless you follow the intent with action then the intent is nothing. For example, I might intend to get fit, but I spend all my time eating pizza and drinking cola as I watch TV. I have my intention, but my actions do not confirm or create the intention. Therefore, if you intend something, do it; don't just talk about it. Action turns knowledge into wisdom.

15. **Freedom of Choice:** We all have free will, and can choose to do anything we wish. There is no situation where we do not have choice. It may appear that we do not, but there are always options as long as we have the courage and strength to take them. We just have to have the courage of conviction to make the decisions.

16. **Change Happens:** Change is continuous and is always happening around us. We cannot actually perceive change, but we can see the end result of it. Change is not a bad thing, and it is not to be feared. Through change we can grow and go forward.

17. **Taking Responsibility:** Our actions cause a reaction—it is a law of nature. We have to be aware of our actions and take responsibility for them and for the consequences of them. It is no good doing something and then saying you did not mean to do it. Had you not meant to do it, you would not have done it. By taking responsibility for our actions, we can take back our power and freedom to choose. We have to accept that no one will live for us and that sometimes our actions will cause others, or ourselves, a measure of discomfort. Remember, though, that feeling discomfort is one way we grow and see where changes need to be made.

18. **One Step at a Time:** To get to any goal, break it down into a number of small steps. If you have many small successes, then this process will lead to a big success. If you aim for a big success straight off, you may fail. Remember that a journey toward any destination

starts with a single step, and then a second and a third, and as many as required until you reach your destination. Remember to reward and praise yourself for your successes, however small they are. By acknowledging them, you increase your power and will to succeed and strengthen your belief in yourself.

19. **Judgment:** We have no right to judge another for their words, thoughts, or deeds. They have the freedom of choice to do as they please and act as they wish, just as we do. We are in no position to judge anyone, as we are imperfect ourselves. It is easy to judge; for example, when you see a big man with tattoos and a shaved head who is wearing leather, your automatic assumption might be that he is trouble. He might be a florist for all you know. Assumptions color our judgment of people and change how we act toward them. By having no preconceptions of other people, you can interact better with them and perhaps make new friends.

20. **Integrity:** Integrity is all about how we act when no one is looking. We must live to our own standards and should not judge others by them. This is about living in line with our highest vision despite urges to the contrary.

21. **Air Your Doubts:** By airing your doubts, fears, and worries—by looking at them and seeing them for what they are—you can conquer them and rid yourself of them forever. When you refuse to confront them, they gain power over you and become even more deeply rooted. After you realize what they are, you can release them.

22. **Failure:** It is very rare for us to fail. We only ever choose to stop trying. That is us exercising our free will. We can stop trying any time we wish, but a person who succeeds never stops until he or she gets to the goal. Success often does not come easy, and it does require work and effort. You will find that most "overnight successes" have been working hard to achieve success for many years. Failure is not something to be feared or worried about because you can never fail! Everything you do, no matter whether you view it as a success or failure, is a valuable lesson to learn. By looking at a perceived failure as a valuable lesson, it no longer feels as bad. The only true failure is not learning the lessons your mistakes teach you.

23. **The Ongoing Journey:** Our journey of exploration through life never, ever stops. The destination is not the reward or the goal. The journey to the destination is the goal itself.

24. **Don't Mind:** If you take an objective view of your mind then you can see that lots of thoughts drift through it, many of which you are unaware of. A sad, angry, or fearful thought may drift up from the subconscious and change how you feel for no apparent reason. You must take control of the mind through tools, such as meditation, and become aware of your thoughts and realize them for what they are. Then, you can let them go and stay relaxed and centered. By consciously focusing on your breathing and keeping it deep and even, you can help to release these negative thoughts.

25. **Emotions:** Emotions come and go. They flow through us all the time, often without us even being aware of it. Many of us do not express our emotions because we feel we have to "be manly" or "be responsible" or "be cool." When we feel the negative emotions, we can feel our bodies tense. If we do not express these emotions when we feel them, the tension is stored within our bodies. Having emotions is not to be feared and should be celebrated. When you feel an emotion, express it! If you are happy, smile and laugh; if you are sad, cry. Expressing your emotions releases the tension they create and helps you live more fully in the here and now. After you have expressed an emotion, it is gone and will not return with the same force for that situation. If you refuse to express your emotions and store them up, eventually the level will rise too high and will overflow, like a river that has been dammed.

26. **Play:** As children, we play exuberantly. We have fun, enjoy ourselves, and have lots of energy. Then something happens; we grow up, and we no longer play. We have a belief that adults have to be "adult," and adults don't play. Playing is one of our greatest sources of pleasure. It takes many forms, from sport to games to laughing and joking with friends. Playing increases our energy and makes us more positive. It makes those around us more positive and generally lifts the spirits of all involved. There are times to be serious, yes, but there are times to play, too, and that is what we must not forget.

# INDEX

## A

AACN (American Association of Critical-Care Nurses), 51

AAMI (age-associated memory impairment), 237

ACOEM (American College of Occupational and Environmental Medicine), 165

Adams, Douglas, 269

Adams, Patch, 218, 223

adaptagenicity, 48–50

adaptogen extracts, antioxidant potential of, 48–49

Adobe Illustrator, 119

Adobe Photoshop, 119

adrenal fatigue/adrenal apathy/adrenal neurasthenia, 145–146

adrenaline and stress, 46

age-associated memory impairment (AAMI), 237

aha moments, 68–69, 70–71, 73

AHNA (American Holistic Nurses Association), 217

AJPH (American Journal of Public Health), 212

Aldefer, Clayton, 11

Allen, James, 41

Allineare, V.L., 234

Amazon
delivery-by-drone, 263
potential time wasters, 137

American Association of Critical-Care Nurses (AACN), 51

American Chiropractic Association, 207

American College of Occupational and Environmental Medicine (ACOEM), 165

American Holistic Nurses Association (AHNA), 217

American Institute of Stress, 54

American Nurses Association (ANA)
fatigue reduction, 147
Nurse Fatigue Panel, 154, 166
Shift Work Disorder Kit, 166

American Psychiatric Association (APA), 222

American Psychological Society, 54

AMI (age-related memory impairment), 237

amino acids, 162
ANA (American Nurses
    Association)
    fatigue reduction, 147
    Nurse Fatigue Panel, 154,
        166
    Shift Work Disorder Kit,
        166
*Anatomy of an Illness as
    Perceived by the Patient,* 218
Android smart phones,
    tablets, and video games,
    smart use of, 127
Angelou, Maya, 69
ANS (autonomic nervous
    system), 101–102
Anthony, Susan B., 16
antibodies IgA/IgB and
    laughter, 216
antioxidant potential of
    adaptogen extracts, 48–49
Any.do, 35
APA (American Psychiatric
    Association), 222
Apple, Inc.
    dreamers changing world,
        80
    technology advancements,
        119
Appleton, Jon, 119
Archimedes, 71–72
*Archives of General
    Psychiatry,* 161
Aristotle, 39
autonomic nervous system
    (ANS), 101–102
Avis car rentals, 77


B

Bacon, Francis, 7
balancing life
    attitude, 270–273

BE, DO, HAVE concept,
    278
    commitments, 28–29
    engagement in life
        flow, 109–110
        presence, 98, 112
    philosophy of 5 Elements,
        32, 275–277
    scorecard, 42–43
    smile therapy, 271
    time for self and others,
        27, 283
    vision boards, 276–277
Baldwin, Christina, 262
bamboo charcoal, 202
Barney, Natalie Clifford, 147
Battle, William, 218
BE, DO, HAVE concept, 278
Beattie, Melody, 276
Bender, Betty, 186
Benner, Dr. Patricia, 255
Birmingham, Carolyn, 221
Bombeck, Erma, 213
Bovine Growth Hormone
    (rBGH), 230
Boxie, 131
Brakeall, Linda, 171
Breath2Relax app, 113
breathing/relaxation
    techniques
    Breath2Relax app, 113
    conducive to dreaming, 89
    conscious breathing, 177
    stress reduction, 59–60,
        106
Brite, Poppy Z., 194
*The British Journal of
    Psychiatry,* depression, sugar
    and carbohydrates, 163
Bryne, Robert, 3
*Bucket List* (movie), 9
bucket lists
    accountability for
        completing, 10

steps for writing, 9
work in progress, 10
Burgess, Anthony, 191
burnout at work, 173–174, 177
Burton, Robert, 218
Byrne, Rhonda, 39

# C

CAFOs (Concentrated Animal Feeding Operations), 230–232
CalenGoo, 34
Cameron, Julia, 280
Canaff, Dr. Audrey, 173
cancer, shift work, 159
Canfield, Jack, 39
cardiovascular diseases
    fatigue, 164
    shift work disorders, 159
CareerBuilder, 173
career changes
    assessment exercises, 245–246
    CareerBuilder, 173
    *Career Reexplosion: Reinvent Yourself in Thirty Days,* 283
    considerations before changes, 250–252, 254–257
    Everybody's Career Company, 246
    greener pastures concept, 259
    multiple changes throughout life, 258–259
    resources available, 257–258
    sharing job enthusiasm, 259–261

treating as adventure, 253–257, 283
*Career Reexplosion: Reinvent Yourself in Thirty Days,* 283
Carlson, Erika, 7
Carson, Rachel, 40
CDC (Centers for Disease Control and Prevention), 191
Cedars-Sinai Medical Center humor study, 222
"Celebration of Spirit," 38
cell phones, dangers, 121–127
Chicago Blackhawks, 79
Chinese medicine. *See* TCM
chitin, 202
Chopra, Deepak, 192
Churchill, Winston, 178
circadian rhythms, 193
Circle of Wellness, 52
cognitive skills
    healthy lifestyles, 237
    MBCT (Mindfulness-Based Cognitive Theory), 97
Cole, Steven, 17
compassion fatigue
    identifying, 157
    interventions, 157–158
    strategies for reducing, 158–159
    symptoms of, 156–157
Concentrated Animal Feeding Operations (CAFOs), 230–232
Conciergist, 35
Confucius, 25
connectivity's impact. *See also* social media/phones/email; technology
    biological damage, 122, 125–127
    on general health, 121
    on hearing, 124

ill effects, current,
122–123, 126–127,
129–130, 136
ill effects, long-term,
125–126
safety tips, 124–125
conscious breathing, 177
Constant Contact,
InfusionSoft, 134
controlled breathing
conducive to dreaming,
89
stress reduction, 59–60,
106
convenience and processed
foods, 234
*Core Curriculum for Holistic
Nursing,* 217
Cousins, Norman, 218
Covey, Stephen, 176
Craigslist, time wasters, 137
Csikszentmihalyi, Mihaly
*Finding Flow: The
Psychology of
Engagement with
Everyday Life,* 113
happiness, 107–108
cybercrime, 120

# D

daily affirmations, 265–266
dairy products, 230
D' Angelo, Anthony J., 117
Davis, Meryl, 79–80
de Balzac, Honoré, 250
DeGeneres, Ellen, 63
dehydroepiandrosterone
(DHEA) levels and
laughter, 216
Delta One stage of sleep, 88
dementia, healthy lifestyles,
237

de Mille, Agnes, 282
de Mondeville, Henri, 218
Department of Agriculture,
U.S., 233
Department of Labor,
U.S., Office of Disability
Employment Policy, 177
depression
EAPs (Employee
Assistance Programs),
55
fatigue, 160
avoiding sugars and
carbohydrates,
162–163
treating vitamin D
deficiencies, 163
treating without drugs,
161–162
learned helplessness
theory, 93
Matt Adler Suicide
Assessment, Treatment
& Management Act,
55
MBCT (Mindfulness-
Based Cognitive
Theory), 97
MBSR (Mindfulness-
Based Stress
Reduction), 97
mental health days, 97
performance costs, 56
shift work, 159
stress symptoms, 48
deprivation of sleep
combating, 203–206
disturbances affecting,
203–206
signs of, 193–194
Descartes, 7
DHEA
(dehydroepiandrosterone)
levels and laughter, 216

Diana, Princess of Wales, 214
Dickinson, Emily, 261
digital technology. *See* technology, digital
Disability Employment Policy, U.S. Department of Labor, 177
diseases, and cell phone use, 123–124
distress *versus* eustress, 47
"Down Memory Lane" game, 265
dreams/dreamers/dreaming
    aids to dreaming
        controlled breathing, 89
        exercise plans, 89
        food/diets, 89
        relaxation/breathing techniques, 89
    defining dreams, 83–84
    engagement in life, 95–96
    examples of, 79–80
    "I Have a Dream" speech, 82
    implementing, 84–85
    importance of, 79
    maintaining, 79–81
    in nursing profession, 82, 86
    supporting, 87–89
    universal dreams, 83
Dropbox, 34, 130
drowsy driving, 154–156
Dr. Phil McGraw, 38
Dr. Seuss, 59
Dweck, Carol S., 274

# E

EAPs (Employee Assistance Programs)
    compassion fatigue, 157–158
    employee assistance from burnout, 177
    stress suffering, 55
Earhart, Amelia, 39
Earth, five elements philosophy, 32, 249–250, 276
eBooks, 130
eco-functional bedding, 207
Edison, Thomas, 84
Edwards, Julie Andrews, 78
Einstein, Albert, 9
electromagnetic fields (EMF)
    connectivity's effects, 126–127
    sleep problems, 203
ELF (extremely low frequency) radiation, 126
EMF (electromagnetic fields)
    connectivity's effects, 126–127
    sleep problems, 203
emotional intelligence, 67, 103
Employee Assistance Programs (EAPs)
    compassion fatigue, 157–158
    employee assistance from burnout, 177
    stress suffering, 55
engagement in life
    assessing, 93
    continuing with dreaming, 95–96
    as default behavior, 94
    definition of, 92

engaged happiness, 92,
107–108
flow, 107–108
assessing, 112
in balance, 109–110
elements of, 108–109
practicing, 112
resources, 112–113
mindfulness
in beginner's minds, 99
in eating, 100–101
meditation, 106–107
nervous systems,
101–103
nonstriving, 103–104
overview of, 99–100
practicing, 112
resources, 112–113
routine practices,
105–106
self-compassion,
103–104
in stress management,
101–103
presence, path to balance,
98, 112
*versus* presenteeism, 55,
96–98
psychological flexibility,
93–95
self-awareness *versus* self-
consciousness, 94–95
Enterprise car rentals, 77–78
EPA (Environmental
Protection Agency), U.S.,
129–130
ERG (Existence/Relatedness/
Growth) Theory, 11, 136
eustress *versus* distress, 47
Evernote, 34, 131
Everybody's Career
Company, 246
exercise plans
conducive to dreaming,
89

impact of, 235
mindfulness, 105–106
stress reduction, 60, 63,
105–106
Existence/Relatedness/
Growth (ERG) Theory, 11,
136
extremely low frequency
(ELF) radiation, 126

# F

Facebook
impact on health, 136
technology overload, 118,
130, 132
time wasters, 34, 137
far-infrared technology
linens, 202
mattresses, 208
fatigue
adrenal fatigue, 145–146
and cardiovascular
diseases, 164
compassion fatigue
identifying, 157
interventions, 157–
158
strategies for reducing,
158–159
symptoms of, 156–157
definition of, 144
and depression, 160
avoiding sugars and
carbohydrates,
162–163
treating vitamin D
deficiencies, 163
treating without drugs,
161–162
effects on performance,
150–155
common effects, 153

drowsy driving,
154–156
on law officers, 153–
154
non-work-related, 149
resulting in injuries,
159–160
safety issues, 152, 154
work-related, 149
and gastrointestinal
problems, 160
mental fatigue, 144–145
and obesity, 163–164
physical fatigue, 145
reduction strategies, 150,
165
alarm management,
159
by all stakeholders,
165
best practices, 151
clear communication,
152
by employees, 149
by employers, 147–
148
FRMS (fatigue
reduction
management system),
165
listening strategies, 178
resources, 166
by systems, 150
wellness environments,
151–152
resources, 166
total fatigue, 146
Fatigue and Hours of Work
Toolkit, 166
fatigue reduction
management system
(FRMS), 165
Fellerman, Hazel, 37
Finding Flow: The Psychology
of Engagement with Everyday
Life, 113

Fire, five elements
philosophy, 32, 249–250,
276
Fitch, Janet, 238
5 Elements of Success, 32,
248–250
5-HTP amino acid, 162
Florida Hospital, 182
flow in engagement in life,
107–108
assessing, 112
in balance, 109–110
elements of, 108–109
practicing, 112
resources, 112–113
focus, 67–68
aha moments, 68–69,
70–71, 73
being centered, 72–73
definition and importance
of, 68–69
discovering passions, 78
dreams/dreamers
defining dreams,
83–84
examples of, 79–80
"I Have a Dream"
speech, 82
implementing, 84–85
importance of, 79
in nursing profession,
82, 86
supporting, 87–89
universal dreams, 83
finding motivation, 75
of life, 70–71
maintaining, 71
dreams, 79–81
focus on main thing,
75–76
setting goals, 77–78
steps for tapping into
creative side, 73
success, result of, 78–79
tipping points, 81

food/diets for healthy living,
225–226, 228
conducive to dreaming,
89
connection to good
health, 225–226, 228
digestion's role, 226–227
at home and away,
226–227
nutrients, 227–228
shopping
CAFOs (Concentrated
Animal Feeding
Operations), 230–
232
convenience and
processed foods, 234
dairy, 230
gluten-free products,
233
GMOs (genetically
modified organisms),
232
halal products, 234
IGF-1 (insulin-like
growth factor), 230
kosher products,
233–234
meat, 230
organic products, 233
produce, 228–229
Proposition 65,
California, 232
rBGH (Bovine Growth
Hormone), 230
vegan products, 233
stress reduction, 56, 61
The Four Agreements, 17
Frank, Anne, 181
Frankl, Victor
finding meaning in suffering,
8
human's attitudes, 272
Franklin, Benjamin
laws of attraction, 39

sleep, 204
Freeman, Morgan, 9
Fried, Barbara, 253
Friedman, Thomas, 20
FRMS (fatigue reduction
management system), 165
Frost, Robert, 197
Fuller, Margaret, 53

# G

gastrointestinal problems
fatigue, 160
role of healthy food/diets,
226–227
shift work, 159
Gates, Bill
dreamers creating change,
80
goal setting, 16
genetically modified
organisms (GMOs), 232
Gesundheit Institute, 218,
223
getAbstract, 34
Getty, John Paul, 184
Ghandi
emulation lives of service,
11
influential people, 9
Gigahertz versus 900 MHz
phones, 124
GL (glycemic load), 163
Gladwell, Malcolm, 81
gluten-free products, 233
GMOs (genetically modified
organisms), 232
goal setting
focus, 77–78
life's purpose, 15–16
elevator speeches, 22
SMART technique, 22
reinventing self, 284
Godin, Seth, 36

Goethe, 84
Goleman, Daniel, 67
Google
    driverless cars, 263
    syncing calendars for
       Android and Apple
       devices, 34
Google+, 137
Graham, Martha, 143
Grappo, Gary Joseph, 283
Gray, Erin, 235
Gray, Theodore, 119
Greer, Germaine, 264
GSP navigation systems, 120
Guidance Statement on
    Fatigue Risk Management
    in the Workplace, 165

## H

Haggerty, Deborah, 270
halal products, 234
Hale, Mandy, 271
Hamilton Rating Scale, 161
Hansen, Grace, 14
Headspace app, 113
"Health Care Worker Fatigue
    and Patient Safety," 144
healthy lifestyles, 212–213
    being merry, 213–214
    emotional energy, 214
    energy-increasing
       guidelines, 215
    exercise and movement,
       impact of, 235
    food/diets
       conducive to
          dreaming, 89
       connection to good
          health, 225–226, 228
       digestion's role,
          226–227
       at home and away,
          226–227

nutrients, 227–228
stress reduction, 56, 61
food shopping
    CAFOs (Concentrated
       Animal Feeding
       Operations), 230–
       232
    convenience and
       processed foods, 234
    dairy, 230
    gluten-free products,
       233
    GMOs (genetically
       modified organisms),
       232
    halal products, 234
    IGF-1 (insulin-like
       growth factor), 230
    kosher products,
       233–234
    meat, 230
    organic products, 233
    produce, 228–229
    Proposition 65,
       California, 232
    rBGH (Bovine Growth
       Hormone), 230
    vegan products, 233
laughing/humor, 211–212
    benefits of, 216–217
    comments to promote,
       221–222
    contagious nature of,
       221, 225
    health benefits of,
       220–224
    laughter yoga, 217
    learning to laugh,
       224–225
    psychology and society
       of, 219–220
    throughout history,
       217–218
    World Laugher Day,
       219

living well, 236
    with agility, 238
    with good balance, 238
    with good cognitive
       skills, 237
    with good memory, 237
    self-awareness test, 239
    without dementia, 237
Hemingway, Ernest, 243
Hepburn, Audrey, 213
Hertz car rentals, 77
Hiero, 71
Hillesum, Etty, 58
Hippocrates, 49
Holford, Patrick, 163
Hootsuite, 34
Howard, Elizabeth Jane, 46
Hui Chen, 32, 275
human needs, 11–12, 136
humor/laughing, 211–212
    benefits of, 216–217
    comments to promote,
       221–222
    contagious nature of, 221,
       225
    health benefits of, 220–221
       example, Cedars-Sinai
         Medical Center,
         220–221
       example, Patch Adams,
         223–224
    laughter yoga, 217
    learning to laugh
       patient care, 225
       work setting, 224–225
    psychology and society of,
       219–220
    throughout history, 217–
       218
    World Laugher Day, 219

# I

ICN (International Council of
    Nurses), 223
ICRW (information-carrying
    radio wave), 126
IGF-1 (insulin-like growth
    factor), 230
"I Have a Dream" speech, 82
IHI (Institute for Healthcare
    Improvement), 182
IM (instant messages), 118
influential people
    characteristics of, 7–8
    identifying, 7–9
information-carrying radio
    wave (ICRW), 126
information overload, 117–118
    connectivity's impact
       biological damage, 122,
         125–127
       on general health, 121
       on hearing, 124
       ill effects, current,
         122–123, 126–127,
         129–130, 136
       ill effects, long-term,
         125–126
       safety tips, 124–125
    social media/phones/email
       controlling, 133–137
       effects on our total
         being, 132–133,
         135–137
       excesses of, 34, 132
       privacy and safety,
         135–137
    technology
       advancement over 30
         years, 119
       cellular, 131–132
       impact on information
         overload, 118

information age
everywhere, 130–131
and privacy, 120
smart use of, 127–128
useful apps, 130–131
wireless, 126–127
InfusionSoft's Constant
Contact, 134
injuries on job, 149, 159–160
instant messages (IM), 118
Institute for Healthcare
Improvement (IHI), 182
Institute of Medicine (IOM),
154
insulin-like growth factor
(IGF-1), 230
International Council of
Nurses (ICN), 223
intuition, trust in, 10–12
basic human needs, 11–12,
136
choices, 12, 16
IOM (Institute of Medicine),
154
iPads/iPhones, smart use of,
127
Islamic dietary laws, 234

**J**

Jackham, Justin, 9
Jefferson, Thomas, 39
Jewish dietary laws, 233
Jobs, Steve, 80
Johnson, Spencer, 256
The Joint Commission (TJC),
"Health Care Worker Fatigue
and Patient Safety," 144
Jones, Karen Sparck, 119
*Just Enough,* 180

**K**

Kant, Immanuel, 218
karma, 40
Kataria, Dr. Madan, 217
Keller, Helen, 76
Key Ring, 34
King, Jr., Martin Luther
dreamers changing world, 9
"I Have a Dream" speech,
82
knowing, center of, and
meditation, 4, 106–107
knowledge *versus* self-
knowledge, 7
Kopp, Wendy, 82
kosher products, 233–234

**L**

Lao Tzu, 4, 29
LastPass, 34
laughing/humor, 211–212
benefits of, 216–217
comments to promote,
221–222
contagious nature of, 221,
225
health benefits of, 220–221
example, Cedars-Sinai
Medical Center,
220–221
example, Patch Adams,
223–224
laughter yoga, 217
learning to laugh
patient care, 225
work setting, 224–225
psychology and society of,
219–220
throughout history, 217–
218
World Laugher Day, 219

laugh out loud (lol) therapy, 218
Laughter Therapy, 218
Lawrence, T.E., 107
Laws of Life, 38–39
    of abundance, 41
    of attraction, 39–40, 42
    of intention, 40
*Lead the Field*, 259
Learning Project program, 82
Lennon, John, 87
life
    analysis of habits, 35
    balancing
        attitude, 270–273
        BE, DO, HAVE
            concept, 278
        commitments, 28–29
        Philosophy of Five
            Elements, 275–277
        scorecard, 42–43
        smile therapy, 271
        time for self and others,
            27, 283
        vision boards, 276–277
    complexities of, 26
    engagement in (*See*
        engagement in life)
    expectancy, QALE
        (quality-adjusted life
        expectancy), 212
    handling change, 274–275,
        278
        changing choices, not
            habits, 281–282
        changing practices, 280
        creating future, 280–281
        shifting paradigms,
            279–280
    Laws of Life, 38–39
        of abundance, 41
        of attraction, 39–40, 42
        of intention, 40
    mindless consumption, 33
    mind-set, 273–274

quantum leaps, 36–38
simplifying, 25
    apps available, 34–35
    enough concept, 31–32
    "Simplify by Five"
        concept, 30–31
    25 principles of, 285–290
life's purpose
    alignment with purpose,
        19–21
    being on purpose, 14–15
    happiness plans, 17–19
    identifying, 4
        meditation's role, 4
        reasons for, 4
        simple approach, 5–6
        through bucket lists,
            9–10
        through circumstances,
            8, 17
        through influential
            people, 8–9
        time requirements, 5–6
        by trusting intuition,
            10–12
    maintaining, 6
    purpose formula, 13
    reimagining, 12–13
    setting goals, 15–16
        elevator speeches, 22
        SMART technique, 22
Lingzhi/Ganoderma/Reishi
    mushroom, 236
LinkedIn, time consumed on,
    34
listening strategies, 178
living longer
    healthy food/diets
        conducive to dreaming,
            89
        connection to good
            health, 225–226, 228
        digestion's role, 226–227
        at home and away,
            226–227

nutrients, 227–228
stress reduction, 56, 61
healthy food shopping
    CAFOs (Concentrated
        Animal Feeding
        Operations), 230–232
    convenience and
        processed foods, 234
    dairy, 230
    gluten-free products,
        233
    GMOs (genetically
        modified organisms),
        232
    halal products, 234
    IGF-1 (insulin-like
        growth factor), 230
    kosher products, 233–
        234
    meat, 230
    organic products, 233
    produce, 228–229
    Proposition 65,
        California, 232
    rBGH (Bovine Growth
        Hormone), 230
    vegan products, 233
laughing/humor, 211–212
    benefits of, 216–217
    comments to promote,
        221–222
    contagious nature of,
        221, 225
    health benefits of,
        220–224
    laughter yoga, 217
    learning to laugh,
        224–225
    psychology and society
        of, 219–220
    throughout history,
        217–218
    World Laugher Day, 219

living well, 236
    with agility, 238
    with good balance, 238
    with good cognitive
        skills, 237
    with good memory, 237
    self-awareness test, 239
    without dementia, 237
lol (laugh out loud) therapy,
    218
Lost, TV show, 109
low-awareness living, 5
The Low-GL Diet Bible, 163

# M

Macintosh computers, 119
Mailbox, 131
Mandela, Nelson
    emulation lives of service,
        11
    recognizing changes in self,
        259
Man's Search for Meaning, 8
"The Man Who Thinks He
    Can," 37
Maslow, Abraham, 11, 136
Matt Adler Suicide Assessment,
    Treatment & Management
    Act, 55
Mayo Clinic, recommended
    sleep, 196
MBCT (Mindfulness-Based
    Cognitive Theory), 97
MBSR (Mindfulness-Based
    Stress Reduction), 97
MBTI (Myers-Briggs Type
    Indicator), 248
McGraw, Dr. Phil, 38
MCI (mild cognitive
    impairment), 237
Mead, Margaret, 72

meat purchases, 230
meditation
   engagement in life, 106–107
   role in life, 4
mental health, definition of, 95
Meron, Neil, 9
metabolic syndrome, 159
Metal, five elements
   philosophy, 32, 249–250, 276
Meyers, Joyce, 277
Michelangelo, 16, 39
Microsoft Corporation, 16, 80
mild cognitive impairment (MCI), 237
Miller, Shannon, 80
Milne, A.A., 58
*The Mindful Brain,* 103
Mindfulness-Based Cognitive Theory (MBCT), 97
Mindfulness-Based Stress Reduction (MBSR), 97
*A Mindfulness-Based Stress Reduction Workbook,* 107, 112
Mindfulness Daily app, Inward, 113
*Mindfulness for Beginners,* 101
mindfulness in life's engagement
   in beginner's minds, 99
   in eating, 100–101
   meditation, 106–107
   nervous systems, 101–103
   nonstriving, 103–104
   overcoming barriers, 7
   overview of, 99–100
   practicing, 112
   resources, 112–113
   routine practices, 105–106
   self-compassion, 103–104
   in stress management, 101–103

Mindfulness Meditation app, 113
Mitty, Walter, 95–96
Mizener, Wilson, 195
moon shots concept, 263
Mother Teresa, 173
   burnout, 173
   emulation of lives of service, 11
   value of smiles, 272
Mozart, Wolfgang Amadeus, 16
mushrooms, medicinal
   longevity, 236
   stress, 49–50
Myers-Briggs Type Indicator (MBTI), 248

N

Nash, Laura, 180
National Academy of Sciences, 17
National Highway Traffic Safety Administration (NHTSA), 156
National Institute for Occupational Safety and Health, 54–55
National Institute of Health, Fact Sheets on Vitamin D, 163
National Security Agency (NSA), 131
National Sleep Foundation Patient Education Portal, 166
National Spelling Bee, 69
National Transportation Safety Board (NTSB), accidents
   drowsy driving, 155
   fatigue-related, 154
National Woman Suffrage Association, 16

negative ion properties, 202
nervous systems
    ANS (autonomic nervous
      system), 101–102
    PNS (parasympathetic
      nervous system),
      101–103
    SNS (sympathetic nervous
      system), 101–103
NetWeaving concept, 189
New Life Solutions, 62
*New Passages,* 253
Newton, Issac, 39
NHTSA (National
  Highway Traffic Safety
  Administration), 156
Nicholson, Jack, 9
Nightingale, Earl, 259
Nightingale, Florence
    dreamers creating change,
      82
    emulation of lives of
      service, 11
    influential people, 9
    theory of nursing, 52
NIH (National Institute of
  Health), Fact Sheets on
  Vitamin D, 163
900 MHz *versus* Gigahertz
  phones, 124
non-Addison's hypoadrenia. *See*
  adrenal fatigue
nonrapid eye movement
  (NREM) stage of sleep, 88
Norwegian University of
  Science and Technology
  (NTNU), 222
NREM (nonrapid eye
  movement) stage of sleep, 88
NSA (National Security
  Agency), 131
NTNU (Norwegian University
  of Science and Technology),
  222

NTSB (National
  Transportation Safety Board),
  accidents
    drowsy driving, 155
    fatigue-related, 154
nutrients, 227–228

## O

Obama, Barack, 79
obesity
    fatigue, 163–164
    shift work, 159
Olympic competitions, 79–80
omega-3 fats, 161
1Password, 131
organic mattresses, 208
organic products, 233
Orr, Leonard, 177
oxidative stress, 49

## P

Palmer, Keke, 149
parasympathetic nervous
  system (PNS), 101–103
*Patch Adams,* movie, 218
performance
    depression costs, 56
    fatigue, 150–155
      common effects, 153
      drowsy driving, 154–
       156
      on law officers, 153–154
      non-work-related, 149
      resulting in injuries,
       159–160
      safety issues, 152, 154
      work-related, 149

*Rise of Superman: Decoding the Science of Ultimate Human Performance,* 113
personal relationships
    ranking in life's purpose, 14
    workplace stress, 54
Phelps, Michael, 80
Pinterest
    time consumed on, 34
    time wasters, 137
Plato, 39
PNS (parasympathetic nervous system), 101–103
*Poems That Live Forever,* 37
polysaccharides, 49
*Pooh's Little Instruction Book,* 58
possessions, ranking in life's purpose, 14
presenteeism
    definition of, 55
    *versus* engagement in life, 96–98
Princess of Wales, Diana, 214
processed and convenience foods, 234
produce purchases, 228–229
professional coaching, 257
professional success, ranking in life's purpose, 14
Proposition 65, California, 232
Pulliam, Keshia Knight, 229
Pulsife, Catherine, 187

## Q–R

QALE (quality-adjusted life expectancy), 212
quality-adjusted life expectancy (QALE), 212
radiation and cellular and wireless technologies, 121–128
    ELF (extremely low frequency) radiation, 126
    EMF (electromagnetic fields), 126–127
    ICRW (information-carrying radio wave), 126
    RF (radio frequency) radiation, 122–123
radio frequency (RF) radiation, 122–123
rapid eye movement (REM) stage of sleep, 88
rBGH (Bovine Growth Hormone), 230
RedLaser, 34
Reeve, Christopher, 87
Reichl, Ruth, 211
reinventing self
    beginning new life
        achieving goals, exercise, 284
        balancing aspects of life, 246
        daily affirmations, 265–266
        jobs, 245–248
        professional coaching, 257
        retirement, 247
    career change
        assessment exercises, 245–246
        considerations before changes, 250–252, 254–257
        greener pastures concept, 259

multiple changes
  throughout life,
  258–259
resources available,
  257–258
sharing job enthusiasm,
  259–261
treating as adventure,
  253–257, 283
considerations, 252–253,
  265
identity crisis, 253
new opportunities
  entrepreneurship, 263
  ignoring age restraints,
    264
  networking, 264
  welcoming, 261–263
recognizing
  need, 244
  your personality type,
    248
relaxation/breathing techniques
  Breath2Relax app, 113
  conducive to dreaming, 89
  conscious breathing, 177
  stress reduction, 59–60,
    106
REM (rapid eye movement)
  stage of sleep, 88
resources
  fatigue, 166
  flow, 113
  mindfulness, 112–113
RF (radio frequency) radiation,
  122–123
Rich Site Summary (RSS)
  feeds, 118, 130
*The Rise of Superman: Decoding
  the Science of Ultimate
  Human Performance,* 113
Robbins, Tony, 38
*Rocky,* 62
*Rolling Stone* digital magazine,
  119

Rowling, J.K., 79
RSS (Rich Site Summary)
  feeds, 118, 130
rubberthane mattresses, 208
Ruiz, Don Miguel, 17

# S

safety issues, fatigue, 152, 154
Salzberg, Sharon, 258
Sandberg, Sheryl, 265
Satir, Virginia
  alignment with life's
    purpose, 21
  creativity, 74
Schumacker, E.F., 28
Schweitzer, Albert, 270
Sebold, Alice, 278
*The Secret,* 39
self-awareness test, 239
self-knowledge, 7
Seligman, Martin, 93–94
Sense of Humor
  Questionnaire, Svebak, 222
serotonin syndrome, 162
*The 7 Habits of Highly Effective
  People,* 176
Sheehy, Gail, 253–254
shift work disorder (SWD),
  50–51
shopping for food
  CAFOs (Concentrated
    Animal Feeding
    Operations), 230–232
  convenience and processed
    foods, 234
  dairy, 230
  gluten-free products, 233
  GMOs (genetically
    modified organisms),
    232
  halal products, 234

IGF-1 (insulin-like growth
factor), 230
kosher products, 233–234
meat, 230
organic products, 233
produce, 228–229
Proposition 65, California,
232
rBGH (Bovine Growth
Hormone), 230
vegan products, 233
Sick Building Syndrome,
129–130
Siegel, Daniel, 103
simplifying life, 25
apps available, 34–35
enough concept, 31–32
"Simplify by Five" concept,
30–31
sleep
accessories affecting
linens with helpful
properties, 202
mattresses, 201, 207–
208
pillows, 201
sleep masks, 202
circadian rhythms, 193
cycles of
NREM (non-rapid eye
movement), 192
REM (rapid eye
movement), 192–193
deprivation
combating, 203–206
disturbances affecting,
203–206
signs of, 193–194
environment for
devices, 200
lighting, 199
medicine/supplements,
200, 206, 208
monitors, 200

music, 199
sound, 199–200
health benefits of, 195
improving quality of, 205
necessity of, 194, 206
positions, 203
quality of, 198
recommended hours of,
195–196
schedule interruptions,
200–201
shift work disorders, 159,
196–197, 205
Sleep and Sleep Disorders
website, 166
smile therapy, 271
Smith, Jada Pinkett, 164
SNS (sympathetic nervous
system), 101–103
social media/phones/email. *See
also* connectivity's impact;
technology
biological damage, 122,
125–127
controlling, 133–137
effects on our total being,
132–133, 135–137
excesses of, 34, 132
privacy and safety, 135–137
Socrates, 39
Sony Walkman, 120
Spencer, Herbert, 218
Stevenson, Howard, 180
Stoll, Dr. Andrew, 161
Stowe, Harriet Beecher, 91
St. Peter's Basilica, 16
Strengths, Weaknesses,
Opportunities, Threats
(SWOT) analysis, 245
stress
adaptagenicity, 48–50
adrenaline, 46
American Institute of Stress,
54

ANS (autonomic nervous system), 101–102
cholesterol levels, 50
coping with, 56
depression
    MBSR (Mindfulness-Based Stress Reduction), 97
    stress symptoms, 48
distress or eustress, 47
managing
    mindfulness, 101–103
    *A Mindfulness-Based Stress Reduction Workbook,* 107, 112
physiology of, 46
PNS (parasympathetic nervous system), 101–103
reducing, 56–61
    breathing/relaxation techniques, 59–60, 106
    comments/actions promoting laughter, 221–222
    doing nothing concept, 58
    eating well, 56, 61
    exercise plans, 60, 63, 105–106
    food/diets, 49–50, 56, 61
    good posture, 61, 106
    prioritizing responsibilities, 61
    relaxation/ breathing techniques, 59–60, 89, 106, 113, 177
    resilience, 62–63
    sleep/power naps, 58, 60, 64
    stress management programs, 62

stress reduction studies, 161
SNS (sympathetic nervous system), 101–103
sources of, 46–47
symptoms of, 47–48
in workplace, 46–47, 50–51
    cost of, 53–56
    EAPs (Employee Assistance Programs), 55, 157–158, 177
    lack of necessary skills, 110
    personal relationships, 54
    stress management programs, 62
    wellness initiatives, 51–53, 55–56
success through integrity concept, 32
Svebak's Sense of Humor Questionnaire, 222
SWD (shift work disorder), 50–51
SWOT (Strengths, Weaknesses, Opportunities, Threats) analysis, 245
sympathetic nervous system (SNS), 101–103

## T

T-cells and laughter, 216
TCM (Chinese Medicine), 5 elements, 236, 275
Teach for America, 82
Teach program, 82
technology. *See also* connectivity's impact; social media/phones/email advancement over 30 years, 119

cellular, 131–132
digital
    advancement of, 119–120
    physical safety of, 121–127
impact on information overload, 118
information age everywhere, 130–131
and privacy, 120
smart use of, 127–128
useful apps, 130–131
wireless, 126–127
Templeton, John Marks, 38
Tharp, Twyla, 26
Things 2, 34
third age, 264
30/30, 131
Thomas, Marlo, 192
Thompson, Emma, 33
Thoreau, Henry David
    life's purpose, 21
    privacy *versus* need to know, 120
*The Tipping Point,* 81
TJC (The Joint Commission), "Health Care Worker Fatigue and Patient Safety," 144
Tolstoy, Leo
    changes in self, 244
    engaging life, 95
Tomlin, Lily, 45
Towers Watson healthcare surveys, 51
tryptophan amino acid, 162
Tubman, Harriet, 86
20 Connected Breaths, 177
Twitter
    technology use, 130
    time consumed on, 34
    time wasters, 137

# U–V

UCLA Mindful Awareness Research Center, 112
UMMS (University of Massachusetts Medical School), 212
University of Massachusetts Medical School (UMMS), 212
USDA Organic seal, 233
U.S. Department of Agriculture, 233
U.S. Department of Labor's Office of Disability Employment Policy, 177
U.S. EPA (Environmental Protection Agency), 129–130

vegan products, 233
vision boards, 276–277
vitamin D deficiencies, 163

# W

Water, five elements philosophy, 32, 249–250, 276
Weldon, Fay, 15
wellness environments, 151–152
White, Charlie, 79
White, E.B., 174
Whitman, Harold, 247
WHO (World Health Organization), 129–130
*Who Moved My Cheese,* 256, 274
wiifYOU website, 254
Wilder, Laura Ingalls
    laughter, 226
    simplifying life, 31

Winfrey, Oprah
  dreaming
    creating change, 80
    importance of, 67–68
    positive thinking, 251
    work/life balance, 187
Wintle, Walter D., 37
Wisconsin Hospital
  Association, Fatigue and
  Hours of Work Toolkit, 166
Wood, five elements
  philosophy, 32, 249–250,
  276
Woods, Tiger, 16
Woolf, Virginia, 80
workplace-related issues
  burnout, 173–174
  fatigue, 149
  negotiation, 171–172
  stress, 46–47, 50–51
    cost of, 53–56
    lack of necessary skills,
    110
    wellness initiatives,
    51–53
  work *versus* personal life,
  174
    balancing work/life, 187
    building connections,
    185
    building family-friendly
    environments, 185–
    186
    centering self, 177
    communicating clearly,
    178–179
    counterbalancing work/
    personal life, 188–189
    developing efficiency,
    175
    integrating teams,
    183–184

knowing limitations,
  176–177
leveraging teams,
  184–185
maintaining personal
  interests, 180
managing time, 175
measuring outcomes,
  179–180
reentering workforce,
  186
requesting help, 178
setting priorities, 176
surrounding self with
  good people, 181–183
switching to part-time
  work, 186
trying new activities,
  180–181
World Health Organization
  (WHO), 129–130
World Laugher Day, 219
Wright brothers, 84

# X–Y–Z

Yao Ming, 80
YouTube, 137
Yovanoff, Brenna, 41

ZipList, 34

# Timely Topics for Practicing Nurses

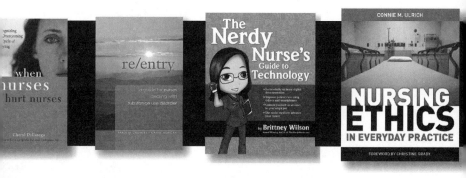

**When Nurses Hurt Nurses:**
Recognizing and Overcoming the Cycle of Bullying

Cheryl Dellasega

**Re-Entry:**
A Guide for Nurses Dealing with Substance Use Disorder

Karolyn Crowley and Carrie Morgan

**The Nerdy Nurse's Guide to Technology**

Brittney Wilson

**Nursing Ethics in Everyday Practice**

Connie M. Ulrich

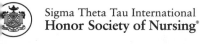
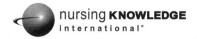

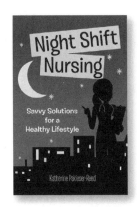
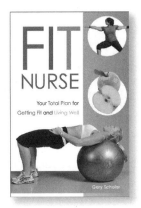
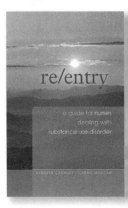
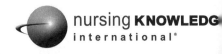